Essential Skills

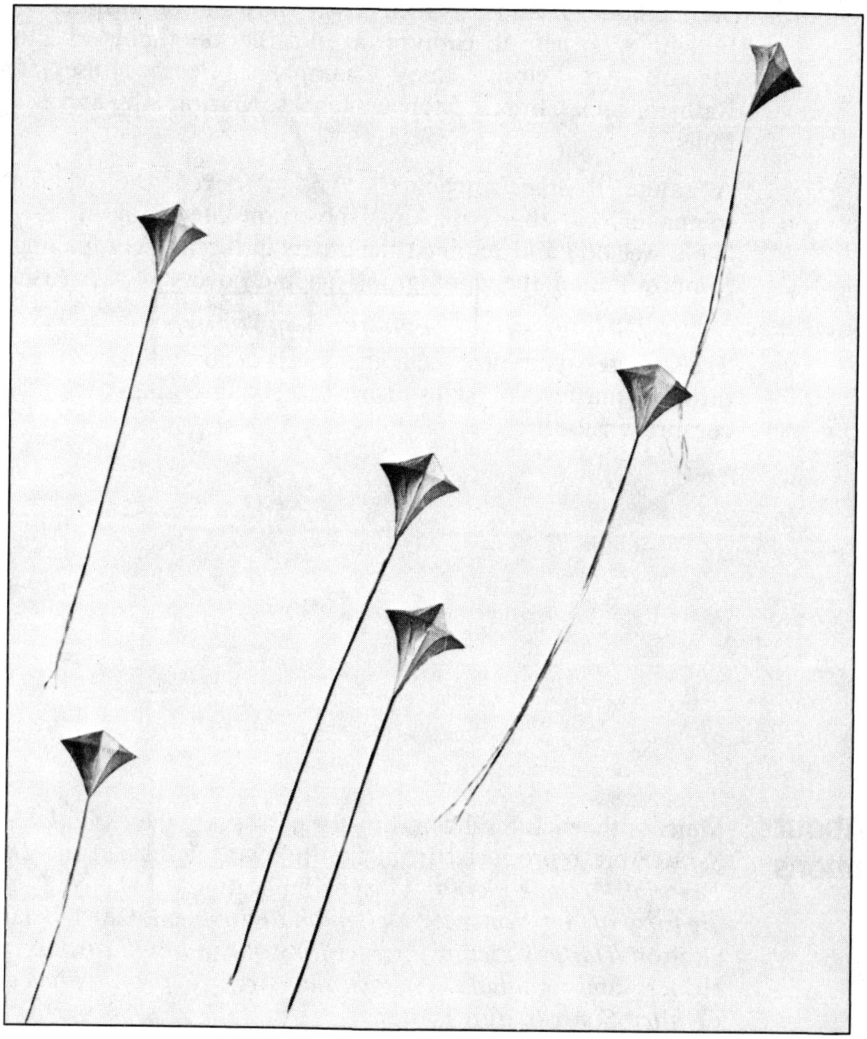

Revised Edition

About the Cover

The breeze was fresh this bright day in May, and gaily-colored kites appeared like spring swallows, darting across the blue sky over Rhode Island's Narragansett Bay. Photographer Tony Botelho was there to capture on film the kite-flights of Christy Menard, Art Pelosi, Danny Champagne, Peggy Hulsey, John Rathjen, Jack Christie, Stephen Jencks, Marion Alig and Megen Mills.

A salute to the rowboaters who retrieved the "diamond-spinnaker" kite that got away! The errant kite shook in the wind like a wet dog and rejoined the others in the sky, completing the composition of the photograph on the covers of the *Essential Skills Series.*

The six kites symbolize the higher levels of comprehension gained through mastery of skills from the six essential categories of comprehension.

About the Illustrations

Many of the pictures illustrating the passages in the *Essential Skills Series* were reproduced from the following books in the *Dover Pictorial Archive Series*, Dover Publications, Inc., New York: *Treasury of Art Nouveau, Design and Ornament*, Carol Belanger Grafton; *Harter's Picture Archive for Collage and Illustration*, Jim Harter; and *Animals: A Pictorial Archive from Nineteenth-Century Sources*, Jim Harter.

Other illustrations are by Howard Lewis and Thomas Ewing Malloy.

Essential Skills Series

Essential Skills

Book 10

Walter Pauk, Ph.D.
Director, Reading Research Center
Cornell University

Revised Edition

Jamestown Publishers
Providence, Rhode Island

Essential Skills Series
No. 310, Book 10

Cover Design by Deborah Hulsey Christie, adapted from the Original Design by Stephen R. Anthony

Text Design by Deborah Hulsey Christie

Printed in the United States of America

8 9 10 11 12 PO 99 98 97 96 95

ISBN 0-89061-229-3

Preface

Practice Makes Perfect

Why do some students shoot baskets over and over again and others skate and reskate the same routine? These beginners know that practice makes perfect. Not only do beginners know this, but pros do too. For what other reason do they work at baseball and football week after week before the opening dates?

Value of Practice

The pros know the value of practice, but they also know the value of something else. They know that practice without *instruction* and *guidance* does not automatically lead to improvement. That's why they have the best coaches that money can buy.

And so it is with developing the skills of reading. There must be the right kind of practicing and the right kind of coaching.

First, a word about practice. In this book the right kind of practice is provided by twenty-five highly interesting and carefully selected passages. Here is material enough on which to grow and keep growing.

Value of Coaching

Now about coaching! Good coaching takes the form of instruction and guidance. In this book the instruction is straightforward and uncomplicated. It puts you directly on the right track, and better still, you are kept on the right track by two unusual systems of guidance. The first system is the uniquely designed, six-way question format which makes sure that every ounce of practice is directed toward improvement. Nothing is wasted!

Diagnostic Chart

The second system of guidance is the Diagnostic Chart. This chart is no ordinary gimmick. In truth, it provides the most dignified form of diagnosis and guidance yet devised. It provides instantaneous and continuous diagnosis and gentle but certain self-guidance. It yields information directly to the student. This form of self-guidance leads to the goal of all education: the goal of self-teaching.

Acknowledgments

Now, I want to make some acknowledgments, especially to the students who were the guinea pigs. Afterwards I told them so, but they said, "We didn't mind even then. And now that it is over, we're all the happier because we know how much we've learned." But what the students did not know was how much I learned from them. For this I thank them all, class after class.

I direct especial thanks to Linda Browning, Anita DuBose, and Karen Duddy for handling the almost countless number of selections, writing and refining the questions and making sure that the series kept moving: all, a most demanding task.

Finally, I am most grateful to authors, editors and publishers who have generously given permission to quote and reprint in this book from works written and published by them. The books quoted in the text and used as sources of reading extracts are listed in the back of the book.

Walter Pauk

Contents

To the Instructor

Selection of Passages

All of us believe in this truism: to learn to read, a person must read. But, placing a book in front of a student won't automatically promote reading.

This last sentence brings up another truism: you can lead a horse to water, but you can't make it drink. To tempt a horse, the water must be clear, cool and clean.

To tempt the student, the passages must be genuinely fascinating. Knowing this, we packed each book with twenty-five "I can't put the book down" type of passages.

Each passage had to meet at least the following criteria: *high interest level, appropriate readability level* and *factual accuracy of contents.* High interest was assured by choosing passages from popular magazines that appeal to a wide range of readers. The readability level of each passage was assessed by applying Dr. Edward B. Fry's *Formula for Estimating Readability,* thus enabling the arrangement of passages on a single grade level within each book. The factual accuracy of the passages is high because they were written by professional writers whose works are recognized and respected.

The Great Value of Questions

Dr. Mortimer J. Adler says that the overall secret for improving one's reading can be boiled down to knowing how to keep awake while reading. He means more than keeping one's eyes open. He means keeping one's mind open and active.

One sure-fire way to do this is to keep trying to answer questions while reading. Questions not only keep one's mind awake, but also keep the mind active, not letting it get flabby. Here's a good story that makes the same point.

> To keep their fish alive for the fresh-fish markets, the owners of fishing boats used a water-filled floating tank. The fish remained alive all right, but they were never firm, always flabby. One captain, however, always brought back firm, fresh, active fish. His fish always received a higher price.

> One day he revealed his secret: "You see," he said, "for every hundred herrings I put into my tank, I put in one catfish. It is true that the catfish eat five or six of the herrings on the trip back to port, but the catfish keep the rest alert and constantly active. That's why my herring arrive in beautiful condition."

The work of the catfish, in this book, is done by the six essential questions (subject matter, supporting details, conclusion, clarifying devices, vocabulary in context, and main idea). These questions keep the minds of students alert, active and in beautiful condition.

The main idea questions in this book are not the usual multiple-choice variety. Given four statements, the students are asked to recognize the main idea of the passage. They also tell why each of the other three does not express the main idea; the students identify one statement as too narrow, one as too broad and one as merely a detail.

By asking these six types of questions in each passage, students quickly learn to read with a questioning and anticipating attitude. This attitude, necessary for high comprehension, is easily transferred to other material such as the textbook.

The Diagnostic Chart

Those who used the first edition of these books had high praise for the Diagnostic Chart. In sum, this is what they said.

> The Diagnostic Chart is truly ingenious because it is, in fact, a self-diagnosing instrument. The Chart instantly, simply and continually shows students their strengths and weaknesses.

Here is how the Chart works. The six questions for each passage are always in the same order. For example, the question designed to teach the skill of making *conclusions* is always in the number three position, and the question designed to teach the skill of identifying *clarifying devices* is always in the number four position, and so forth. This innovation of keeping the questions in order sets the stage for the smooth functioning of the Chart.

The Chart works automatically when the letters of the answers are placed in the spaces on the Chart. Even after completing one passage, the Chart will reveal the type or types of questions answered correctly as well as the types answered incorrectly. But more important, the Chart will identify the types of questions missed consistently. More persuasive identification is possible after three or more passages have been completed. By then, a pattern can be observed. For example, if the answers to question number three (making conclusions) are incorrect for all three passages, or on three out of four, then this weakness shows up automatically.

Once a weakness is revealed, instruct the students to take the following steps: First, turn back to the instructional pages to study the section in which the topic is discussed. Second, go back to read again the questions in that particular category that were missed; then, with the correct answers in mind, read the entire passage again, trying to see how the author developed the answers to the questions. Third, on succeeding passages, put forth extra effort to answer correctly the questions in that particular category. Fourth, if the difficulty still persists, arrange for a conference with the instructor.

To the Student

Understanding the Six Essential Skills

What reading skills do readers need to know to gain meaning from what they read? To gain meaning, readers need to know at least six essential skills. They need to know how to concentrate or focus on the writing. This helps them learn what the subject matter of the writing is. They need to know how to grasp the main idea or point of the writing. They need to know how to draw conclusions based on the facts in the passages. They need to know how to recognize the writer's clarifying devices or methods of making the story clear and alive. And they need to know how to unlock the meaning of the words they encounter. Let's take a closer look at these skills.

Concentration/ Subject Matter

Readers often say, "I can't concentrate!" It's a problem they can't seem to lick. But there is a sure, fast cure. There is no better way to gain concentration when reading than this: after reading the first few lines, ask yourself the question, "What is this passage about?" In other words, "What is the general subject matter?"

If you don't ask this question, here's what will probably happen. Your eyes will move across the lines of print. Yet your mind will be thinking of other things.

But if you ask the question, you will begin to *think*. Once you begin *thinking* about what's being said in the passage, you are then *concentrating*. Let's see if this method works. Here are the first lines of a passage:

> Wood ducks are the most beautiful ducks in North America. Once they were rare. Now — if you have sharp eyes and can keep quiet — you might see them in almost any woodland along streams and ponds.

After reading this, you most likely assumed that the author will talk about the wood duck. Now that your mind is on the trail, the chances are good it will follow the author's idea line by line. Thus, you will *concentrate* on the building of the subject matter.

Let's try the method again. Here are a few lines from another passage:

> Of all the little animals in the world, the Columbian ground squirrel is one of the liveliest and friendliest. It is nicknamed "picket pin" because it sits as stiff and straight as a stake in the ground.

Again, you probably had no trouble picking out the subject matter: the Columbian ground squirrel.

Main Idea

Once the subject matter has been grasped, it is time for the next question. Ask yourself, "What is the author's main idea?" "What point is the passage trying to make?"

With such questions in mind, you can be sure that an answer often pops up. But when no questions are asked, all things seem the same to the reader. Nothing stands out, so the reader will not see the point of the passage.

Let's look at another passage. This time we will find the main idea.

> Wood ducks never nest on the ground as most ducks do, but in a big hole in a tree. Trees with big holes in them are hard to find.

Since you don't have the full passage to read, I will tell you the answer. The main point is that with fewer and fewer old, dead trees with holes in them, we will have fewer and fewer wood ducks.

Thus, when questions are asked, the reader is truly acting upon the content. Reading becomes a two-way street with both reader and writer engaged. In a sense, the reader talks with the author. So the passage comes to life. Reading becomes an exciting and enjoyable experience.

Supporting Details

Do we like details? Of course we do. In longer articles, main ideas and sub-ideas are like the bones of the writing. They are the skeleton of the passage. The details are the flesh. They give the writing fullness and life.

Details are used to support the main ideas. So the term *supporting details* is appropriate. These supporting details come in many forms, but the most common forms are examples, definitions, comparisons, contrasts, repetitions and descriptions.

The author of "The Wood Duck" lets us know that the passage is about wood ducks. Next, the author makes sure we learn the point that without trees with holes, the wood duck will not nest. Thus, there would be fewer wood ducks.

Now that we are interested in this problem, the author gives us details on how we can provide trees with holes in them. The author describes how we can build a wood duck nesting box. Here's the excerpt:

> Why don't you and your parents put up a wood duck nesting box right now? It would be about two feet (about .61 meters) high and ten inches (about 25.4 centimeters) square. Make the entry hole about four inches (about 10.2 centimeters) in diameter. Use rough lumber on the inside, so the ducklings can climb up the sides to the hole. Put wood shavings in the bottom; the mother duck will lay her eggs using these as a nest. To keep her eggs warm, she covers them with her own feathers. If you don't have a tree near the water, you'll need a post. Place the box ten to thirty feet (about 3.1 to 9.1 meters) high.

You can see in the above passage how important details are in telling a story. Details let the reader see what's going on, tell how to do something, how to take action, what something looks like, and so on.

In long passages, there will be some or many sub-ideas. It is important to be careful not to mistake a sub-idea for a main idea. Sub-ideas are broader than details. Still, the sub-ideas are not the main point. The main idea has to do with the whole passage, but the sub-idea has to do with just part of it. Note that in the next example, the sub-idea is about the food that wood ducks eat. The whole passage is *not* about food, so it is *not* the main idea. Usually, you will see that a sub-idea takes the space of one paragraph. Often, the *topic sentence* of the paragraph is a concise statement of a sub-idea.

The following excerpts show how the author groups and structures supporting details around the sub-ideas that are stated in topic sentences. A sub-idea will hold a group of details together.

> Wood ducks like to eat acorns and all kinds of nuts. Their stomachs (or gizzards) have such powerful muscles that they can break the hardest nuts, some that you could barely crack with a hammer! Wood ducks like berries, duckweed and insects. But best of all they like to eat spiders. That's ice cream to them.

The author implies in the topic sentence, the first sentence, that the food which wood ducks like to eat will be discussed. Next, the author describes how the newly hatched ducklings get down to the ground from their nest. Here are more details clustered around another sub-idea:

> Sometimes they nest in holes up in trees that are twice as high as a flagpole. Just think, the baby ducklings must jump to the ground the day they hatch. Usually they don't get hurt, though, because they're light, like little puffs of cotton. The mother stands at the foot of the tree and calls and calls. The ducklings peek out of the hole. Then, like little paratroopers, they jump quickly, one right after the other, to join their mother, who must then hurry them to the pond where they're safe.

Thus, one of the main functions of supporting details is to give some fullness to the passage. The passage would be a rather uninteresting, skimpy statement of one main idea together with its bare-boned sub-ideas if not for details. The details give life to the passage.

Conclusion

As a reader moves through a passage, grasping the main and sub-ideas and their details, it is only natural for the reader to begin to guess an ending or conclusion to the story. Such guesses are part of the sport of reading. Often the author gives the reader an ending. In such a case, the joy of reading lies in the fact that the reader discovers the guess was right. But the conclusion may not be given. The reader then will try to guess the ending which is hinted by the author.

In the excerpts just read about the wood duck, the conclusion takes the form of having the reader see the pleasure of observing a wood duck. The concluding sentence is this:

> If you're lucky, though, and if your (duck) house is in place before the ice melts, you will have a wood duck family in the summer.

In another selection entitled "From Pond to Prairie," the author has this conclusion:

> Finally, there is no longer much open water. The pond has disappeared. Depending on the kinds of plants that have filled it, the pond may be called a bog or a marsh. As changes continue for many more years, the bog may become a forest.

The skillful reader is like a detective. This reader follows the story, always thinking, "Where is the author leading me?" "What is the final point?" "What's the conclusion?" The reader, like a detective, must try to guess the conclusion, changing the guess if necessary as the story unfolds.

Clarifying Devices

The author uses clarifying devices to make the points in the story clear and alive. In a sense, the topic sentence may be thought of as a clarifying device, for it is placed at the start of a paragraph of details. This opening position gives the reader a quick point of focus. The point of the passage becomes clear after reading the topic sentence.

But more often, by clarifying devices, we mean the literary devices in the passage. These are words or phrases which make the ideas, sub-ideas and details clear and which keep them in order.

Authors use literary devices to provide interest and vividness. An example of such a device is the *metaphor,* as in "But best of all they like to eat spiders. *That's ice cream to them.*" This metaphor makes the passage real to the reader. It compares something the reader knows and takes pleasure in — ice cream — with the pleasure ducks get out of eating spiders. The imagination of the reader is brought to bear on the passage. Again, the reader becomes active in the story and actually takes part in it by comparing known experiences with those encountered in reading.

Another literary device which works the same way is the *simile,* a metaphor beginning with "like" or "as." "Like little paratroopers, they (the ducks) jump quickly, one right after the other, to join their mother" is a simile. It is fun to imagine the little ducks copying the activity of paratroopers jumping from a plane.

Besides metaphors and similes, other clarifying devices are organizational patterns. One common pattern is to unfold the events in the order of time. Thus, one thing happens first and then another and another, and so forth.

The time pattern orders the related event. The event may take place in the span of five minutes or five centuries. A time pattern may be used to describe the habits of an animal from its birth to its death.

You should learn to recognize these literary devices. They help you to understand the passage and speed your reading. They allow you to participate in your reading.

Vocabulary in Context

A reader who does not know what the author's words mean may not understand the passage. Certainly, the reader should look up the unknown words in a dictionary.

In addition, a reader may know only the general meaning of the word. But sometimes a more exact meaning is needed to grasp the passage more fully. A reader who places a general meaning on a word may end up with a blurred picture of the idea. An exact meaning will give the reader a full and clear picture.

For instance, in the next excerpt are two common words many people feel they already know. Consequently, they don't see the need to look them up in the dictionary. But few people know the exact meanings of these words.

> Depending on the kinds of plants that have filled it, the pond may be called a *bog* or a *marsh.*

Do you know the difference between a bog and a marsh? Is there a difference? If so, what is it? How would your mental picture change if you knew?

Looking up words for their exact meanings is rewarding. A precise vocabulary leads to better understanding.

You may find it troublesome to look up words you feel you already know, but you should get into this habit to improve your reading. Of course, words you do not know must always be looked up. You would most likely need a dictionary for these words:

> Nothing could appear more *benign* than a field aglow with daisies, goldenrod and Queen Anne's lace.

> *Sphinxlike,* it crouches among the flowers until the desired insect wanders within reach.

The dictionary is like a stock market. Here you exchange fuzzy meanings for exact meanings. And you get new meanings for unknown words. All this is at no cost other than a flip of your finger.

Answering the Main Idea Question

Being able to find the main idea of everything you read is one of the most important reading skills you can develop. To develop this skill is one aim of this book. The main idea questions in the *Essential Skills Series* are not the usual multiple-choice questions. Instead, each main idea question is made up of four statements. Two of the statements refer to only parts of the passage. One of these is a *detail.* It states a detail that has little bearing on the article as a whole. The other statement is *too narrow*. It tells more than the detail statement, but it's too specific to tell about the main point of the passage.

The last two statements deal with the entire passage. One is *too broad*. It is too general and too vague to be a good main idea statement.

The remaining statement is the *main idea*. It tells *who* or *what* the subject of the passage is. The main idea statement also answers the question *does what?* or *is what?*

Read the sample passage below. Then follow the instructions in the box. The answer to each part of the main idea question has been filled in for you, as well as the score for each answer.

Sample

Tangled in a wire fence, the coyote struggled to get free. Its leg was cut and bruised. The pain must have been terrible. But the animal never stopped trying to get loose.

Two young farm girls saw the trapped coyote. They hurried to a nearby house. The farmer heard their story and came to help.

They held the coyote's head in place with hoe handles. Then they cut the wire fence. The coyote slipped free. But the animal stood still. Perhaps it wanted to thank its rescuers.

The animal had to be gently nudged before it would leave. At last it hobbled off. Then it turned, pausing to look again at the good people who had saved its life.

		Answer	Score
Mark the main idea	. . . .	M	10
Mark the statement that is a detail	. . . .	D	5
Mark the statement that is too narrow	. . . .	N	5
Mark the statement that is too broad	. . . .	B	5

a. **Two young girls helped to free a trapped coyote.**
[This statement is a summary that gathers all the essential points to give an accurate picture of the main idea in a brief way: (1) two young girls, (2) a trapped coyote, and (3) freeing it.] M 10

b. **Kind hearts set free a doomed coyote.**
[This statement is too general. It doesn't state *who* set the coyote free or *why* it was doomed.] B 5

c. **Hoe handles were used to hold the coyote's head.**
[This is only one of many details mentioned in the passage. It has little to do with the passage as a whole.] D 5

d. **A wire fence was cut to set a coyote free.**
[Cutting the fence is *part* of the main idea. But any main idea statement must give the chief actors credit. It must include the two girls who were responsible for saving the coyote's life.] N 5

The following steps could be called "tricks of the trade." Your teachers might call them "rules for learning." It doesn't matter what they are called. What does matter is that they work.

Think About the Title

An internationally famous linguist told me a "trick" to use every time I read. "The first thing to do is to read the title. Then spend a few moments thinking about it."

Writers spend considerable time thinking up good titles. They try to pack a lot of meaning into them. It makes sense, then, for you to spend a few seconds trying to determine the significance. These few moments of thought will give you a head start on a passage.

Thinking about the title can help you in another way, too. It helps you concentrate on a passage before you actually begin reading. Why does this happen? Thinking about the title fills your head so full of thoughts about the passage that there's no room for anything else to enter to break concentration.

The Dot System

Here is a step that will speed up your reading and improve comprehension at the same time.

After spending a few moments with the title, read *quickly* through the passage. Then, without looking back, answer the six questions by placing a dot in the box beside each answer of your choice. The dots will be your "unofficial" answers. For the main idea question (question six), place your dot in the box alongside the statement that you think is the main idea.

The dot system helps by making you work harder on your first, *fast* reading. The practice you gain by trying to grasp and retain ideas makes you a stronger reader.

The Check-Mark System

After you have answered all of the questions with a dot, read the passage again, *carefully*. This time, make your final answer to each question using a check mark (✓). Read each question. Then place a check mark in the box next to the answer of your choice. The answers with the check marks are the ones that will count toward your score.

To answer the main idea question, follow the special instructions given on each question page. Use a capital letter to indicate your final answer to each part of the main idea question.

The Diagnostic Chart

Now transfer your final answers to the Diagnostic Chart on page 102. Use the column of boxes under number *1* for the answers to the first passage. Use the column of boxes under number *2* for the answers to the second passage, and so on.

Write the letter of your answer in the *upper* portion of each block.

Correct your answers using the Answer Key on pages 100 and 101. When scoring your answers, do *not* use an *x* for *incorrect* or a *c* for *correct*. Instead, follow this method. If your answer is correct, make no mark in the lower part of the answer block. If your answer is *in*correct, write the letter of the correct choice in the *lower* part of the block.

Properly used, then, the answer column for each passage will show not only your incorrect answers, but also the correct answers.

Your Total Comprehension Score

Go back to the passage you have just read. If you answered a question incorrectly, underline the correct response on the question page. Then write your score for each question in the circles provided. Add the scores to determine your Total Comprehension Score.

Graphing Your Progress

After you have computed your Total Comprehension Score, turn to the Progress Graph on page 103. Write your score in the box under the number for each passage. Then put an *x* along the line above the box to show your Total Comprehension Score. Join the *x*'s as you go; plot a line showing your progress.

Taking Corrective Action

Your incorrect answers give you a real opporunity for self-teaching. Take the time to study your wrong answers.

Go back to the original question and read the correct answer (the one you have underlined) several times. With the correct answer in mind, go back to the passage itself. Read to see why the approved answer is better. Try to see where you made your mistake. Try to figure out why you chose a wrong answer.

The Steps in a Nutshell

Here's a quick review of the steps to follow in order to get the most out of each *Essential Skills* book. Be sure you have carefully read and understood all of the information in the "To the Student" section (pages 11 through 22) before you begin.

1. **Think About the Title of the Passage.** Try to get all the meaning the writer put into it.
2. **Read the Passage Quickly.**
3. **Answer the Questions, Using the Dot System.** Use dots to indicate your unofficial answers. Don't look back at the passage.
4. **Read the Passage Again — Carefully.**
5. **Mark Your Final Answers.** Put a check mark (✓) in the box to indicate your final answer. Use capital letters for each part of the main idea question.
6. **Transfer Your Answers to the Diagnostic Chart.** Record your final answers in the upper blocks of the chart on page 102.
7. **Correct Your Answers.** Use the Answer Key on pages 100 and 101. If an answer is incorrect, (a) write the correct answer in the lower block, underneath your wrong answer; and (b) go back to the original question and underline the correct answer.
8. **Calculate Your Total Comprehension Score.** Find your Total Comprehension Score by adding up the points you earned for each question.
9. **Graph Your Progress.** Record and plot your scores on the graph on page 103.
10. **Take Corrective Action.** Study your wrong answers. Read the passage again and try to figure out why you were wrong.

Passages and Questions

Titles of Passages

1. Life in Total Darkness

Have you ever wondered what you would eat if there were no green plants? No corn or potatoes or wheat for bread? There wouldn't be any meat or milk either because cows and all other animals depend directly or indirectly on green plants. There wouldn't be fish because even in water, tiny green plants are the basis of the "food chain."

But everyone knows that green plants grow only where there is light. In the underworld of caves there is only darkness and, therefore, no green plants. If that is true, and it is except in electrically lighted caves, where do cave animals get the food which supplies the energy to keep them alive?

There are two ways. Bats, rats, salamanders and some cave crickets and spiders may leave the cave at night. They eat outside the cave. Often they return before they have digested their meal. The excrement or *guano* of bats and even of insects, such as cave crickets, builds up in thick layers in some caves.

This becomes a food supply for the animals which don't come out, the ones which live in darkness forever. Scientists call them *troglobites* (TRAH gloh bites), true cave dwellers. Most of them would die quickly from sunstroke or sunburn if carried out of the cave in daytime. They have no pigment in their skins to keep out the sun's harmful rays. Their skins are white and so thin that the animals would dry up and die except in a very damp place.

Some have no eyes at all; others have very small eyes but no optic nerves. Either way they are totally blind. What use would eyes be to them in the dark? They have developed other means of finding their way and food.

White cave fish live in many of the cave streams. They are totally blind but are definitely sensitive to even the slightest disturbance. Most of these fish have vibration receptors along their heads and sides of the body which detect movement in the water and guide the fish to their prey. If a cave cricket, a fly or even a mosquito splashes into the water, the blind fish investigates.

Because fish and crayfish that live outside caves move swiftly and sometimes wildly, they use up much energy. But the white, blind cave dwellers move slowly. Their swimming seems effortless and this pays big dividends. They have lower energy use and so less need for food "fuel." This efficiency — getting more "go to the gallon" — may not seem important. But don't forget that there is much less food in a cave than outside, where plant life is the basis of the food supply.

?

	Possible Score	Your Score
1. This passage mainly discusses ☐ a. cave creatures. ☐ b. underground streams. ☐ c. the food chain. ☐ d. limestone caverns.	15	
2. What is the basis of our "food chain"? ☐ a. Green plants ☐ b. Vitamins ☐ c. Minerals ☐ d. Bacteria	15	
3. A person who is always moving or active ☐ a. has a lesser need for energy. ☐ b. uses a great deal of energy. ☐ c. does not need much food. ☐ d. is storing energy.	15	
4. The writer introduces this passage by ☐ a. being comical. ☐ b. making a list. ☐ c. giving a command. ☐ d. asking questions.	15	
5. Harmful rays are ☐ a. gentle. ☐ b. dangerous. ☐ c. electrical. ☐ d. helpful.	15	

6. Main Idea

	Answer	Score
Mark the main idea	M	10
Mark the statement that is a detail	D	5
Mark the statement that is too narrow	N	5
Mark the statement that is too broad	B	5

a. Animals in totally dark caves can still get food to live.

b. Fish in dark caves eat insects which fly into the cave.

c. The white, blind cave-dwelling fish move slowly.

d. Some animals have limited food supplies but manage to survive.

Total Comprehension Score
(Add your scores and enter the total on the graph on page 103.)

Categories of Comprehension Questions

No. 1: Subject Matter	No. 4: Clarifying Devices
No. 2: Supporting Details	No. 5: Vocabulary in Context
No. 3: Conclusion	No. 6: Main Idea

2. Charge!

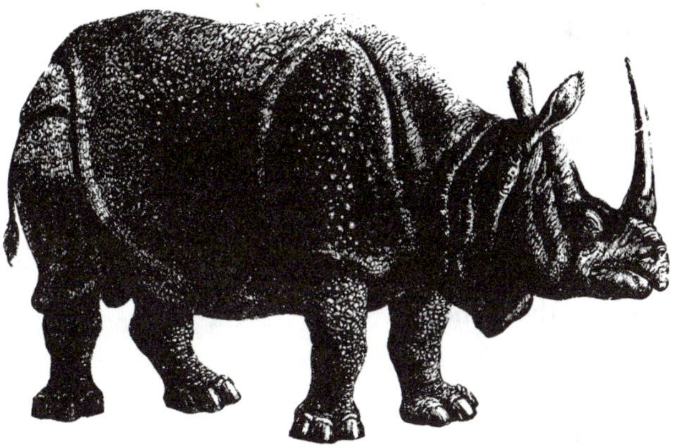

The ill-tempered rhino has a keen sense of smell and an acute sense of hearing, but its eyesight is exceedingly dim. Some people have suggested that its nervous temper results from its nearsightedness — that it charges from fear and uncertainty. However, its rare cousin, the white or square-lipped rhino, is just as myopic, and the white rhino is as docile as a barnyard cow.

If nothing else, the black rhino's poor eyesight leads to frequent clashes with people. While an elephant or buffalo will spot people some distance away and move off, a rhino is not aware of their presence until they are almost upon it, and then trouble often follows.

The rhino's fury is directed against inanimate objects as well. Often it will charge a car and, by dashing it with its great horns, reduce someone's four-wheel pride and joy to junk. One Kenya game warden who found a rhino stuck in a mud hole pulled it out with a Land Rover. The rhino repaid the favor by bashing in the side of the vehicle. On another occasion, a rhino in Kenya was seen battering furiously at a parked tractor. Indeed, the rhinos sometimes charge passing trains. But this is an uneven match, and the train wins.

The black rhino's bad temper is such that it is even conceived in a rage. If a female feels amorous, she charges headlong at a likely suitor and bashes and gores him until he is a bloody mess. If, after this, the male is still willing — and, of course, still alive — mating takes place. The deed done, the female may then batter the male a few more times for good measure.

After eighteen months of gestation, a bouncing sixty-pound (about 27.2-kilogram) baby is born. Twins are unknown. The calf suckles until it is about two years old. By the time it is five to seven years old, it is fully grown and goes off to live by itself. Black rhinos lead a solitary existence all their lives. If two bulls meet, they occasionally battle until one or both are dead.

?

	Possible Score	Your Score
1. Most of this passage talks about ☐ a. the family life of the rhinoceros. ☐ b. where the rhino lives. ☐ c. the nature of the black rhinoceros. ☐ d. the white or square-lipped rhino.	15	
2. The gestation period for the rhino is ☐ a. 6 months. ☐ b. 1 year. ☐ c. 18 months. ☐ d. 2 years.	15	
3. We can infer that rhinos live alone because ☐ a. there are too few left to form a herd. ☐ b. they do not like to share their food. ☐ c. they do not get along with each other. ☐ d. it is easier to escape danger when alone.	15	
4. How did the Kenya game warden feel after the rhino repaid the kind deed? ☐ a. Helpful ☐ b. Regretful ☐ c. Cheerful ☐ d. Hopeful	15	
5. A docile rhino is ☐ a. bold. ☐ b. violent. ☐ c. discontented. ☐ d. gentle.	15	

6. Main Idea

	Answer	Score
Mark the main idea	M	10
Mark the statement that is a detail	D	5
Mark the statement that is too narrow	N	5
Mark the statement that is too broad	B	5

a. Black rhinos live alone. ☐ ◯

b. The black rhino is bad tempered. ☐ ◯

c. The black rhino is so bad tempered it might charge a car. ☐ ◯

d. Where black rhinos are, trouble often follows. ☐ ◯

Total Comprehension Score
(Add your scores and enter the total on the graph on page 103.) ☐

Categories of Comprehension Questions

No. 1: Subject Matter	No. 4: Clarifying Devices
No. 2: Supporting Details	No. 5: Vocabulary in Context
No. 3: Conclusion	No. 6: Main Idea

3. The Snowy Egrets

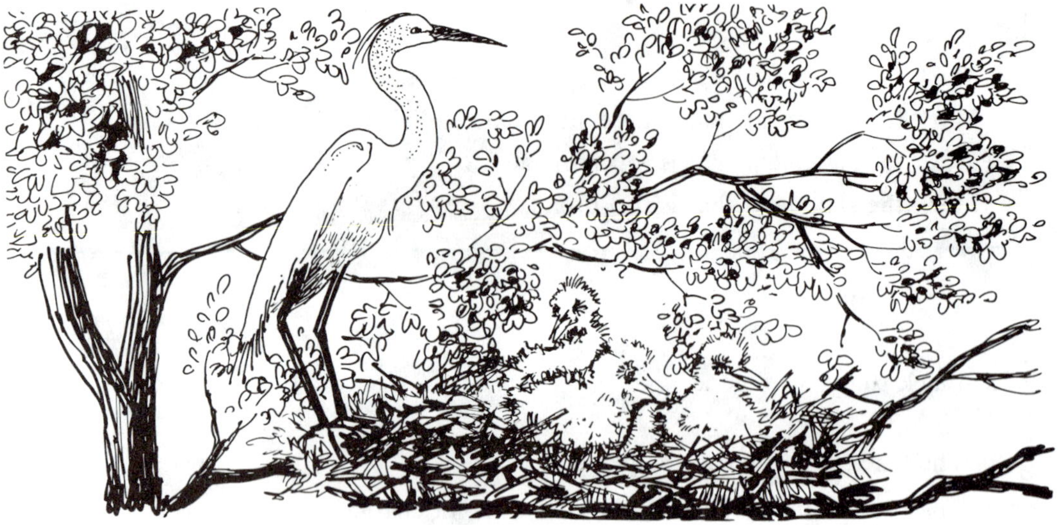

What beautiful birds the snowy egrets are! Some are twenty-four inches (about 61 centimeters) tall. Their feathers are pure white. Their shiny, black bills and legs and their bright yellow feet stand out against their pretty white plumage.

Did you know that the beautiful plumes of the snowy egrets almost caused them to disappear from the earth? Well, during the 1890s, ladies liked to wear the fluffy egret feathers on their hats, so the birds were killed by the thousands. Baby birds were left either starving or unhatched in their shells.

But a young man named Edward McIlhenny decided that the birds must be saved. He filmed the horrible killing of the egrets and the plight of their starving young and toured the country speaking to school children and their parents. He also went to Washington, D.C., to speak to the lawmakers in the United States Capitol.

Then he learned of a rich Indian prince who built cages for birds he had captured to please his young bride. Long after the cages had fallen to pieces, the birds that had been raised in those cages still returned to the same site to nest. Without wasting any time, Mr. McIlhenny went into the Louisiana swamps and caught seven young snowy egrets. He placed them in a large cage built over part of a lake and watched them grow. That fall he let the egrets go and saw them disappear over the Gulf of Mexico, heading south toward their faraway wintering places. He wondered if they would return to the lake where they could be protected and allowed to raise their young without danger.

Did they? Yes, the egrets returned to the cages, and the colony at Bird City started to grow. The Bird City sanctuary is now one of the largest colonies of snowy egrets in the entire world.

?

	Possible Score	Your Score
1. The snowy egrets are ☐ a. white mice. ☐ b. a type of dog. ☐ c. cats. ☐ d. birds.	15	
2. Snowy egrets were hunted for ☐ a. their plumes. ☐ b. food. ☐ c. their eggs. ☐ d. their nests.	15	
3. This passage hints that ☐ a. the egrets never returned to the lake. ☐ b. people can help animals survive. ☐ c. animals do not like cages. ☐ d. the Bird City sanctuary no longer exists.	15	
4. The writer feels that egrets are ☐ a. shy. ☐ b. good to hunt. ☐ c. clever. ☐ d. beautiful.	15	
5. As used in this passage, a <u>plight</u> is ☐ a. an easy way to eat. ☐ b. a difficult situation. ☐ c. a promise. ☐ d. a healthy appearance.	15	

6. Main Idea

	Answer	Score
Mark the main idea	M	10
Mark the statement that is a detail	D	5
Mark the statement that is too narrow	N	5
Mark the statement that is too broad	B	5

a. Since egrets returned to the same nest each year, they multiplied. ☐ ◯

b. Edward McIlhenny saved the snowy egrets from extinction. ☐ ◯

c. The Bird City sanctuary is one of the largest colonies of snowy egrets. ☐ ◯

d. Humans have saved certain animals from extinction. ☐ ◯

Total Comprehension Score ☐
(Add your scores and enter the total on the graph on page 103.)

Categories of Comprehension Questions

No. 1: Subject Matter	No. 4: Clarifying Devices
No. 2: Supporting Details	No. 5: Vocabulary in Context
No. 3: Conclusion	No. 6: Main Idea

4. Timber Wolf

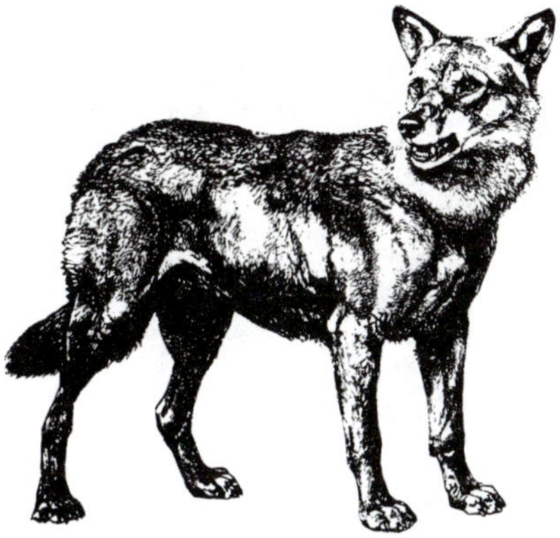

At one time there were more than two million timber wolves. They roamed over almost all of North America. They lived in close family groups called *packs*. They hunted deer, moose, caribou and rabbits for food.

Then the settlers came. They cut down the forests and killed much of the wildlife the wolves needed for food. The wolves found the settlers' livestock easy prey and began killing it for food.

The settlers declared a war on the wolves. This war lasted until just a few years ago. Today only about 800 timber wolves survive in the United States outside of Alaska. Almost all of them live along the border of Minnesota and Canada. More and more people are becoming concerned that the wolves may die out altogether. They are now protected as an endangered species.

To protect the wolves and help them increase in number, we must learn much more about them. Scientists are trying an experiment. They want to return wolves to some of the areas they lived in just a few years ago.

This kind of wolf "transplanting" may cause problems — not because of the wolves, but because of people. Many people believe wolves hurt or even eat people. This is not true. No one has been able to prove that a healthy wolf has ever attacked a human.

Many people still believe another story about wolves — that wolves kill too many animals. But like other meat-eating animals, wolves prey mainly on old, crippled or diseased animals. This leaves the healthier animals to live in balance with their environment.

?

	Possible Score	Your Score
1. The timber wolf is ☐ a. very dangerous. ☐ b. an endangered species. ☐ c. very shy. ☐ d. a problem to ranchers.	◯	15
2. Wolves live in family groups called ☐ a. clans. ☐ b. herds. ☐ c. flocks. ☐ d. packs.	◯	15
3. The wolf seems to be ☐ a. misunderstood by people. ☐ b. a poor hunter. ☐ c. easy to tame. ☐ d. moving south.	◯	15
4. The first paragraph tells us how wolves ☐ a. get their food. ☐ b. make their homes. ☐ c. are killed. ☐ d. lived in the past.	◯	15
5. What is a wolf's prey? ☐ a. The place a wolf lives ☐ b. A wolf's family ☐ c. The animal it captures and eats ☐ d. The kind of fur it has	◯	15

6. Main Idea

	Answer	Score
Mark the main idea	M	10
Mark the statement that is a detail	D	5
Mark the statement that is too narrow	N	5
Mark the statement that is too broad	B	5

a. Many animals which help nature are nearly extinct.

b. Wolves are nearly extinct animals which help balance nature.

c. Today only about 800 timber wolves live in the lower United States.

d. Wolves live in close family groups.

Total Comprehension Score
(Add your scores and enter the total on the graph on page 103.)

Categories of Comprehension Questions

No. 1: Subject Matter	No. 4: Clarifying Devices
No. 2: Supporting Details	No. 5: Vocabulary in Context
No. 3: Conclusion	No. 6: Main Idea

5. The Grasshopper Hunter

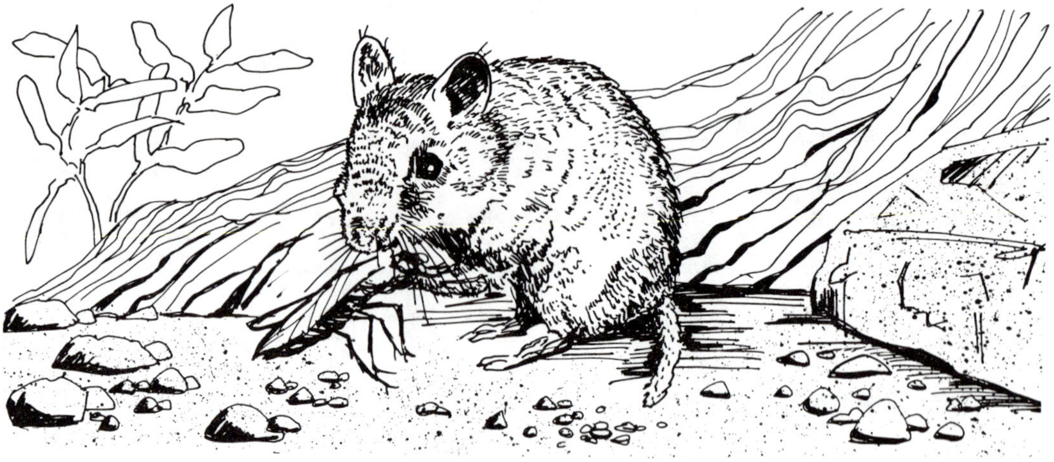

The boiling heat of the day at last begins to leave the desert sand. Soon stars will dot the sky. The animals which have hidden underground since early morning come out of their cool daytime hideaways.

A giant cactus stands tall over the desert. Its many branches reach for the sky like spiny arms. An elf owl, hidden safely within, peers out of its hollowed-out home high in the big cactus.

A long, sharp whistle breaks the stillness like a tiny wolf howl. Somewhere nearby a plump little mouse stands on its hind legs and throws back its head. With its mouth wide open, the mouse gives its strange cry again.

Then the mouse is off, searching through the night. With its nose to the ground, the little hunter starts its nightly search for food.

Suddenly its step quickens. Hot on the trail now, whiskers shaking, the mouse scurries closer to its prey. A final rush and . . . *pounce*! A surprised grasshopper finds itself tightly held in the mouse's front paws. After a quick bite into the grasshopper's head, the little mouse sits up on its haunches, holds the prey in its front paws and daintily nibbles away.

And so it goes, all through the desert night. The grasshopper was only a snack to the hungry mouse. The mouse will eat much more before the night is over.

This mouse is different from other kinds of mice, which eat mostly seeds or grasses. This little mouse likes to eat grasshoppers, crickets, beetles and other insects — and this is why it is called the grasshopper mouse. The grasshopper mouse will often dig up juicy larvae or insect eggs which it has found with its keen sense of smell. It also eats lizards, toads and even scorpions, but only after biting off the scorpion's poisonous stinger. In fact, the grasshopper mouse eats so many scorpions that in Colorado it is known as the *scorpion mouse.*

?

	Possible Score	Your Score
1. This passage talks about the ☐ a. kangaroo rat. ☐ b. field mouse. ☐ c. scorpion mouse. ☐ d. white mouse.	15	
2. The grasshopper mouse eats mostly ☐ a. small cacti. ☐ b. dead animals. ☐ c. seeds. ☐ d. insects.	15	
3. The grasshopper mouse gets its prey by ☐ a. trapping it. ☐ b. hunting it. ☐ c. waiting for it. ☐ d. playing a trick on it.	15	
4. A "plump little mouse" is ☐ a. pretty. ☐ b. thin. ☐ c. weak. ☐ d. fat.	15	
5. As used in this passage, peer means to ☐ a. look. ☐ b. run. ☐ c. scream. ☐ d. crawl.	15	

6. Main Idea

	Answer	Score
Mark the main idea	M	10
Mark the statement that is a detail	D	5
Mark the statement that is too narrow	N	5
Mark the statement that is too broad	B	5

a. The grasshopper mouse hunts insects, lizards, toads and even mosquitoes.

b. The grasshopper mouse will eat scorpions after biting off the stinger.

c. The grasshopper mouse has a long, sharp whistle.

d. Not all mice eat seeds and grasses.

Total Comprehension Score
(Add your scores and enter the total on the graph on page 103.)

Categories of Comprehension Questions

No. 1: Subject Matter	No. 4: Clarifying Devices
No. 2: Supporting Details	No. 5: Vocabulary in Context
No. 3: Conclusion	No. 6: Main Idea

6. The Jackass Penguin

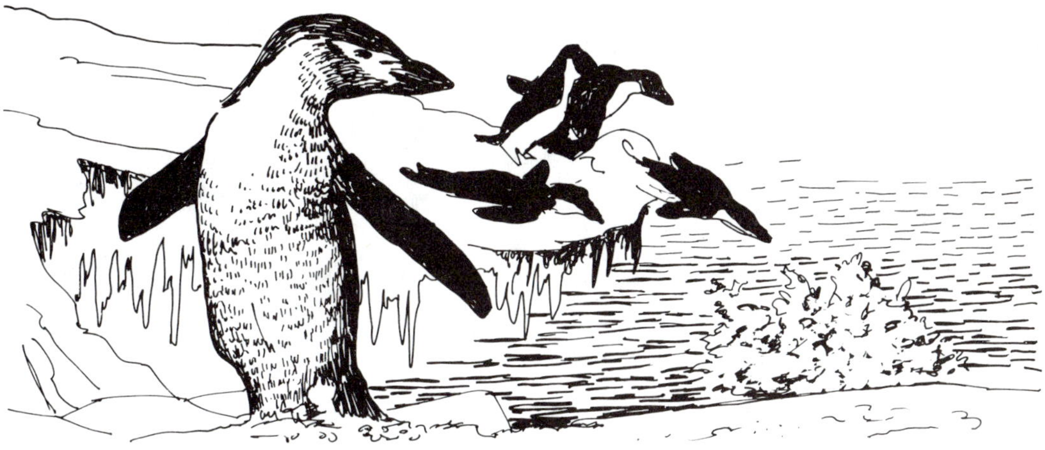

If you should visit the southern coast of South Africa someday, don't be surprised if a small black and white bird, standing straight up, waddles right up to you. It might even "hee-haw" at you. If it does, you will have met the jackass penguin.

Portuguese sailors with Vasco da Gama, the explorer, were the first Europeans to report seeing these funny birds. In 1498 Vasco da Gama and his men sailed around the Cape of Good Hope at the tip of South Africa. They returned with stories about creatures "about the size of ganders, with a cry resembling the braying of jackasses."

These early explorers weren't exactly sure what the animals were. Nobody had ever heard of a bird that could swim as well as these creatures did. They looked like birds, but had "flippers" and swam like seals.

Many years later, scientists discovered that what the sailors had seen were penguins, true birds that had lost the ability to fly.

Most jackass penguins are found at the Cape of Good Hope. The coastline where they live is very hot and dry, but jackass penguins don't spend much time on land. The water, which is cooled by the current coming up from the Antarctic, is their favorite place!

The feathers on the wings of penguins are short, close together and waterproof, making their wings more like flippers. The jackass penguins are small compared to the large emperor penguins, which sometimes are four feet (about 1.2 meters) tall. The little African penguins usually stand about twenty-eight inches (about 71.1 centimeters) tall, no taller than an umbrella.

Like all kinds of penguins, the jackasses always live in groups. These huge groups live in colonies called *rookeries.* Each mated pair of penguins digs its own nesting burrow on the bare shore. The scooped-out hole is filled with sticks, grass and seaweed. The penguins will use the same nest as long as they live.

?

	Possible Score	Your Score
1. The jackass penguin is a ☐ a. small black and white bird. ☐ b. large hunting fowl. ☐ c. type of duck. ☐ d. desert bird.	15	
2. Where are these penguins found? ☐ a. Portugal ☐ b. Cape of Good Hope ☐ c. Northern Spain ☐ d. Antarctica	15	
3. Unlike some birds, the jackass penguin seems to nest ☐ a. on steep cliffs. ☐ b. in caves. ☐ c. in short bushes. ☐ d. on the ground.	15	
4. The writer of this passage compares the wings of the penguin to ☐ a. arms. ☐ b. branches. ☐ c. legs. ☐ d. flippers.	15	
5. A nesting <u>burrow</u> is ☐ a. a hole in the ground. ☐ b. a rock shelter. ☐ c. a nest made of twigs. ☐ d. a small pool of water.	15	

6. Main Idea

	Answer	Score
Mark the main idea	M	10
Mark the statement that is a detail	D	5
Mark the statement that is too narrow	N	5
Mark the statement that is too broad	B	5

a. The jackass penguin amazed early explorers. ☐ ○

b. Jackass penguins have flippers and can swim like seals. ☐ ○

c. Jackass penguins are unusual African birds which bray like jackasses. ☐ ○

d. The jackass penguin stands about 28 inches (about 71.1 centimeters) tall. ☐ ○

Total Comprehension Score
(Add your scores and enter the total on the graph on page 103.) ☐

Categories of Comprehension Questions

No. 1: Subject Matter	No. 4: Clarifying Devices
No. 2: Supporting Details	No. 5: Vocabulary in Context
No. 3: Conclusion	No. 6: Main Idea

7. Danger Afloat

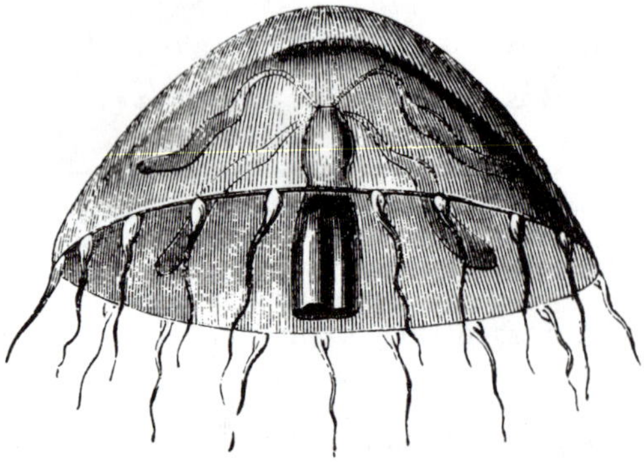

If after a storm you ever see a beach covered with objects that look like small, bright-blue, plastic pillows, step carefully. They could be Portuguese men-o-war. Even if they are dead, their tentacles pack a walloping sting that may make you miserable for days.

The Portuguese men-o-war usually stay in the warm waters of the Gulf Stream. But sometimes these jellyfish are blown onto the Atlantic shores of the United States and Europe.

Their balloon-like blue "floats," filled with gas, are carried along easily by the wind. The float itself is topped by a crest like the sail on a sailboat. The crest can be raised or lowered when the man-o-war wants to move fast or slow. It is not visible when the man-o-war is feeding.

Sailors of long ago thought the crest looked like a sail on a Portuguese fighting ship. Because of this, they gave the jellyfish the name Portuguese man-o-war. Jellyfish are still known by this name.

A man-o-war is not one animal, but a colony of animals called *polyps* (POLL ips). They are all joined to the hollow float, and carried along by it. Each polyp has a different job to do: some reproduce, others protect the colony, and a third group finds food. The polyps look like a brown and pink mass directly under the float.

Stringlike tentacles hang down from the float and act like arms. These tentacles may drift as far as 100 feet (about 30.5 meters) below the surface of the water. Any small fish that is unlucky enough to swim into this drifting forest of "string" is caught in the tentacles and paralyzed by stinging cells. The fish is then pulled up and eaten.

Swimmers in warm waters would be wise to stay away from these floating jelly fish. Human victims say they felt as if they had been "attacked by a swarm of angry bees."

?

1. The Portuguese man-o-war is

	Possible Score	Your Score
☐ a. a squid. ☐ b. a jellyfish. ☐ c. an octopus. ☐ d. a starfish.	15	

2. The Portuguese man-o-war is usually found

☐ a. in the Gulf Stream. ☐ b. near the Arctic. ☐ c. in the Pacific Ocean. ☐ d. in the Mediterranean Sea.	15	

3. The writer hints that after a storm many Portuguese men-o-war are

☐ a. found in underwater caves. ☐ b. hidden in deep water. ☐ c. washed ashore. ☐ d. able to find more food.	15	

4. Stringlike tentacles would be

☐ a. short and thick. ☐ b. long and thin. ☐ c. white and bony. ☐ d. a large soft ball.	15	

5. The crest on the Portuguese man-o-war is sometimes <u>visible</u>. This means

☐ a. the crest is soft. ☐ b. it can sting. ☐ c. the man-o-war is colorful. ☐ d. it can be seen.	15	

6. Main Idea

	Answer	Score
Mark the main idea	M	10
Mark the statement that is a detail	D	5
Mark the statement that is too narrow	N	5
Mark the statement that is too broad	B	5

a. Be careful around Portuguese men-o-war whether they are on beaches or in the water. ☐ ○

b. The tentacles may drift as far as 100 feet (about 30.5 meters) below the surface of the water. ☐ ○

c. Portuguese men-o-war are animal colonies which have stinging tentacles. ☐ ○

d. The stinging tentacles paralyze small fish, which are then pulled up and eaten. ☐ ○

Total Comprehension Score ☐
(Add your scores and enter the total on the graph on page 103.)

Categories of Comprehension Questions

No. 1: Subject Matter	No. 4: Clarifying Devices
No. 2: Supporting Details	No. 5: Vocabulary in Context
No. 3: Conclusion	No. 6: Main Idea

8. A House With Legs

If you could look far, far back in time, you would see a world much different from our world today. Strange creatures would be crawling, creeping or jumping about in a steamy, tropical swamp. Very few would look familiar to you. But you would recognize the turtle.

Fossil remains show that this kind of creature lived even before dinosaurs roamed the earth. Turtles have changed very little in 200 million years.

People have never been able to figure out how these gentle, awkward reptiles have lasted so long on earth. The turtle's unusual skeleton probably has something to do with it. The turtle lives inside the largest part of its skeleton — its shell. This is its "house with legs," as well as its defense in some cases.

There are many kinds of turtles around the world. There is the young, two-inch (about 5.1 centimeter), red-eared turtle that is sold in pet stores. The giant leatherback sea turtle can grow up to eight feet (about 2.4 meters) long and weigh as much as 1,200 pounds (about 544.4 kilograms). But they are all a great deal alike.

Of what is the house roof made? The top of the turtle is called a *carapace* (KAR uh pace). Depending on the kind of turtle, the carapace may be slightly or greatly arched; it may be smooth or rough; it may be plain or patterned.

Like all good roofs, it has two layers. The inner layer is bone formed from overgrown, widened ribs coming out of the turtle's spine. The outer layer is a series of horny plates of material like that in hooves, horns, claws or your own fingernails. There are two exceptions: The softshell turtle and the leatherback have an outer layer of tough "leathery" skin.

Does the house have a floor? It does, but a very strange one! It is called the *plastron.* Like the roof, it also has two layers, but in this case they are both horny growths and quite smooth. Since there are no walls, the floor and roof curve toward each other and meet along the sides.

If one turtle could envy another, all other kinds would surely envy the box turtle. It is the *only* turtle that can completely pull its head, neck, legs and tail into its house and tightly close it all around.

With other turtles the floor is sometimes not quite as wide as the roof so these turtles can't pull themselves in all the way and close up. This leaves much of the underside of its neck, legs and even a part of its body unprotected. Should this kind of turtle get flipped over on its back by a predator, it becomes a tasty meal.

?

	Possible Score	Your Score
1. What is this passage mostly about? ☐ a. The alligator turtle ☐ b. Turtle shells ☐ c. Turtle eggs ☐ d. Young turtles	15	
2. The bony top of the turtle is called the ☐ a. arch. ☐ b. spiracle. ☐ c. plastron. ☐ d. carapace.	15	
3. Which of the following seems to be true? ☐ a. A turtle uses its shell for protection. ☐ b. Turtles appeared on earth after the dinosaurs. ☐ c. The box turtle does not have a shell. ☐ d. Many people have leatherback turtles as pets.	15	
4. A steamy, tropical swamp would be ☐ a. rocky and lifeless. ☐ b. dry and empty. ☐ c. sandy and windy. ☐ d. very hot and wet.	15	
5. <u>Envy</u> has to do with ☐ a. happiness. ☐ b. jealousy. ☐ c. fighting. ☐ d. sadness.	15	

6. Main Idea

	Answer	Score
Mark the main idea	M	10
Mark the statement that is a detail	D	5
Mark the statement that is too narrow	N	5
Mark the statement that is too broad	B	5

a. The turtle has an unusual skeleton.

b. The box turtle is protected more completely than other turtles.

c. The turtle's shell is designed for housing and protection.

d. Giant leatherbacks can weigh 1,200 pounds (about 544.4 kilograms).

Total Comprehension Score
(Add your scores and enter the total on the graph on page 103.)

Categories of Comprehension Questions

No. 1: Subject Matter	No. 4: Clarifying Devices
No. 2: Supporting Details	No. 5: Vocabulary in Context
No. 3: Conclusion	No. 6: Main Idea

9. What Makes A Bird A Bird?

It is not the laying of eggs that makes a bird a bird because some reptiles lay eggs that look very much like birds' eggs. Even two mammals, the strange duckbilled platypus and the spiny anteater of Australia, lay eggs.

It is not the ability to sing that makes a bird a bird since many mammals can sing and some birds cannot sing at all. What, then, makes a bird?

The one thing that all birds have that no other animals have is feathers. Feathers are of different sizes, shapes and colors. They grow from little pits in the skin. You can see these pits on a chicken or turkey before it goes into the oven.

How long ago did animals with feathers exist? When did feathers first appear? Nobody knows. We do know that a creature that lived in what is now Bavaria, Germany, about 150 million years ago had feathers almost exactly like those found on birds today. Scientists call this creature *Archaeopteryx* (ar kee OP ter ix), from two Greek words meaning "ancient wing." Three fossils of Archaeopteryx have been found in layers of limestone. This limestone was at one time very fine silt or mud at the bottom of a shallow sea. The bodies of the three Archaeopteryx must have fallen into the water. They were covered by the mud at the bottom, and when the mud hardened, the skeletons became fossilized. From these fossils, scientists judge that the Archaeopteryx was about the size of a crow.

These skeletons are so much like reptile bones that scientists probably would have believed they belonged to lizardlike animals, except for one thing. All three fossils show the imprints of feathers, so we must call Archaeopteryx a bird.

Was Archaeopteryx the first bird? Not exactly. It is the oldest one we know about, but it already had feathers. Thus, the ancestor of these birds must have lived even longer ago than 150 million years. We think this ancestor was probably a reptile that lived in trees and jumped from branch to branch. Long flat scales at the edges of the arms helped the animal keep its balance in the air and, like a parachute, slowed down its fall if it missed a branch. Scientists believe that over millions of years these scales changed. They became lighter and more flexible and grew farther back from the edge of the arm. Eventually the scales became feathers and the arms became wings.

Perhaps someday the scientists who study fossils, the *paleontologists* (pay lee on TOL uh jists), will find a fossil that will show us how feathers came to be. All we know now is that such an animal must have lived more than 150 million years ago, before Archaeopteryx sailed through the air with its modern-looking wings.

?

	Possible Score	Your Score
1. This passage explains how birds ☐ a. keep their bodies warm in winter. ☐ b. build their nests. ☐ c. fly through the air using air currents. ☐ d. are different from other animals.	15	
2. Archaeopteryx was fossilized in layers of ☐ a. shale. ☐ b. limestone. ☐ c. volcanic ash. ☐ d. marble.	15	
3. The first bird probably looked more like a ☐ a. reptile. ☐ b. fossil. ☐ c. amphibian. ☐ d. marsupial.	15	
4. "Fossilized skeletons" are the ☐ a. soft fleshy parts of an animal. ☐ b. remains of stored food. ☐ c. bony remains of an animal. ☐ d. remains of ancient eggs.	15	
5. Silt is ☐ a. stone. ☐ b. hair. ☐ c. mud. ☐ d. lava.	15	

6. Main Idea

	Answer	Score
Mark the main idea	M	10
Mark the statement that is a detail	D	5
Mark the statement that is too narrow	N	5
Mark the statement that is too broad	B	5

a. All birds have feathers.

b. The Archaeopteryx had feathers, so it was a bird.

c. Archaeopteryx lived 150 million years ago.

d. Birds are distinct from other creatures.

Total Comprehension Score
(Add your scores and enter the total on the graph on page 103.)

Categories of Comprehension Questions

No. 1: Subject Matter	No. 4: Clarifying Devices
No. 2: Supporting Details	No. 5: Vocabulary in Context
No. 3: Conclusion	No. 6: Main Idea

10. The Lion's Full Bloom

At the top of the dandelion's root, at ground level, is a "secret" — the deeply notched leaves. These leaves spread out in a circle, or *rosette,* and do a good job of preventing needed sun from reaching other plants, such as grass. These leaves may also choke or crowd out any nearby growth.

When the plant is growing in a place where it is not likely to be harmed, the leaves may be well above ground level at the tips. But take a look at a dandelion growing where the lawn mower has a regular route. The leaves lie close to the ground, and the lawn mower hardly touches them.

Up from the center of the plant rise one, two or even several hollow stems. They carry a plentiful supply of moisture to the top of the dandelion. As you may have noticed, these stems stand up proud and strong as long as they are attached to the plant. But, if you break them off, they become limp, saggy strings within a few minutes. The moisture drains out of them very quickly. If you have ever tried to make a bouquet of dandelion blossoms, you know they will not last. Now you know why.

Next we come to another "secret", the one that is the most amazing part of the dandelion. This is the charming yellow blossom, or *head.* We may call it a flower, but it is really a tight cluster of many flowers. Dandelions are members of a group of plants called *composites* (come PAHZ its). Each little, bright golden "petal" in a dandelion bloom is actually a complete flower in itself, able to form a seed. Called a floret, it does its part to make sure that new dandelions will continue to grow. The dandelion is a tough, healthy plant that is definitely built for survival.

?

Question	Possible Score	Your Score

1. What would be another good title for this passage?

   ☐ a. How to Get Rid of Weeds
   ☐ b. Make a Dandelion Salad for a Change
   ☐ c. What Makes a Dandelion?
   ☐ d. Seeds to Sell

   Possible Score: 15 — Your Score: ◯

2. Each little flower on the blossom of the dandelion is called a

   ☐ a. flout.
   ☐ b. florist.
   ☐ c. florin.
   ☐ d. floret.

   Possible Score: 15 — Your Score: ◯

3. Dandelion flowers become very limp when they do not receive

   ☐ a. nitrogen.
   ☐ b. sunlight.
   ☐ c. water.
   ☐ d. carbon dioxide.

   Possible Score: 15 — Your Score: ◯

4. A rosette is

   ☐ a. square.
   ☐ b. round.
   ☐ c. triangular.
   ☐ d. rectangular.

   Possible Score: 15 — Your Score: ◯

5. Notched leaves have

   ☐ a. thick edges.
   ☐ b. lacey edges.
   ☐ c. a smooth, unbroken edge.
   ☐ d. cuts on the outer edges.

   Possible Score: 15 — Your Score: ◯

6. Main Idea

	Answer	Score
Mark the main idea	M	10
Mark the statement that is a detail	D	5
Mark the statement that is too narrow	N	5
Mark the statement that is too broad	B	5

a. The dandelion flower is really many flowers together. ☐ ◯

b. The dandelion is built for survival. ☐ ◯

c. The dandelion's leaves, stem and blossom do their part to help it survive. ☐ ◯

d. A dandelion's leaves prevent sun from reaching nearby plants. ☐ ◯

Total Comprehension Score
(Add your scores and enter the total on the graph on page 103.) ☐

Categories of Comprehension Questions

No. 1: Subject Matter	No. 4: Clarifying Devices
No. 2: Supporting Details	No. 5: Vocabulary in Context
No. 3: Conclusion	No. 6: Main Idea

11. The Protective Parent

As soon as possible after birth, a fawn is moved to an area where there is good, low vegetation for protective cover. Numerous observers have reported watching a doe "talk" its fawn down before leaving it. When the fawn persisted in following, the doe would press it down with her foot. Once down it would remain hidden when the doe departed.

During the first few days of life, its main protection is in staying hidden. When danger is around, it will press flat upon the ground with its head and neck extended and ears laid back against its neck. In this way it becomes a very inconspicuous mound with the many small spots looking like little sunspots on a log. A fawn only a few days old will remain this way until picked up. After about five days, it is steady enough afoot to bound off at the last moment.

The doe remains nearby. Upon the approach of any type of danger, except human, she makes an appearance and decoys it away. If this doesn't work, she will vigorously defend her young with sharp, powerful hoofs.

Another protective mechanism in effect the first few days of a fawn's life is that it is scentless. On many occasions dogs that are known to track deer have been seen to pass within a few feet (about a meter) of a fawn without showing any sign of recognition. Associated with the scentlessness is the fact that the doe stays away from the fawn, returning to nurse and wash it eight to ten times a day.

A doe's milk is very rich, having about three times the butterfat and protein as that of a Jersey cow. At two or three weeks, the fawn starts to supplement its diet with tender vegetation. Although it may appear to eat sufficient natural food at two months, it has been demonstrated that fawns deprived of milk at this age will not survive. A fawn will be three months before it is independent of its mother's milk, though it may continue to nurse another month when permitted.

One of the myths about fawns is that they will be abandoned if touched by humans. This is not so. Human scent around a deer range is common enough that it is of little cause for concern to the doe.

?

	Possible Score	Your Score
1. The main subject of this passage is ☐ a. a deer farm. ☐ b. a young deer. ☐ c. deer hunting. ☐ d. an old stag.	15	
2. Doe's milk is rich in ☐ a. butterfat. ☐ b. calcium. ☐ c. iron. ☐ d. minerals.	15	
3. A doe will fight ☐ a. for her food. ☐ b. in captivity. ☐ c. when her young are threatened. ☐ d. if her mate is in danger.	15	
4. The author compares the fawn's coat to ☐ a. sunspots on a log. ☐ b. polka dots. ☐ c. a canvas covering. ☐ d. a leopard's fur coat.	15	
5. An inconspicuous mound is ☐ a. easy to find. ☐ b. moist and muddy. ☐ c. well hidden. ☐ d. empty.	15	

6. Main Idea

	Answer	Score
Mark the main idea	M	10
Mark the statement that is a detail	D	5
Mark the statement that is too narrow	N	5
Mark the statement that is too broad	B	5

a. A doe nurses its fawn 8 to 10 times a day. ☐ ○

b. The doe will protect the fawn by decoying intruders away. ☐ ○

c. Animal babies survive in different ways. ☐ ○

d. The fawn is protected from danger in several ways. ☐ ○

Total Comprehension Score
(Add your scores and enter the total on the graph on page 103.) ☐

Categories of Comprehension Questions

No. 1: Subject Matter	No. 4: Clarifying Devices
No. 2: Supporting Details	No. 5: Vocabulary in Context
No. 3: Conclusion	No. 6: Main Idea

12. The Robin

When the first English settlers went to North America, they saw in the meadows and woodlands a familiar red-breasted bird. They listened to its beautiful song and watched as it built its nest close to their cabins and began to raise a family.

This bird reminded them of the robin redbreast they had known so well back home in England, so they gave it the same name, "robin." It was a good name for this common North American bird because it is much like its English cousin. They are both members of the thrush family. The main difference between them is size: the six-inch-long (about 15.2-centimeter-long) English robin is a little more than half the size of its North American relative.

The English robin is found all over Europe and in North Africa. But only in England is it more friendly to humans than the North American robin usually is. Everywhere else in Europe, robins are more likely to be birds of the wild woodland areas.

In England the robin stays around the yard throughout the year. Each male bird has its own territory which it defends against all other robins. At my home in Buckinghamshire, England, my bird feeder is on the dividing line between the territories of two robins. Some fierce battles take place over the feed I put out for them.

When spring comes, the soft flowing song of the male soon attracts a female and only then are two birds seen together. They build their small nest in a box or even in an old tin can. Each year one of "my" robins nests in the birdhouse under the cherry tree. It catches small, green caterpillars from under the leaves to feed its hungry young ones.

When the young birds first learn to fly, they are so tame that they sometimes fly right into the house for food. They have speckled breasts. It is not until they are several months old that they get their lovely, red breast feathers.

Halfway around the world another group of English people settled. Remembering their familiar robin redbreast at home, they, too, named a bird "robin" because it looked like the one they had left behind in England. This is the so-called red-capped robin of Australia. It isn't a member of the thrush family at all, but a member of the flycatcher family! It is very small and has the most brightly colored red breast of all the robins — and a red cap to match.

There are many other robins found throughout different parts of the world. Be on the lookout next time you travel abroad.

?

	Possible Score	Your Score
1. What would be another good title for this passage? ☐ a. Mating Time Is Near ☐ b. Help! Save the Robin ☐ c. Robins of the World ☐ d. A Sign of Spring	15	
2. The red-capped robin of Australia is a member of the ☐ a. thrush family. ☐ b. flycatcher family. ☐ c. quail family. ☐ d. sparrow family.	15	
3. We can guess that male and female robins are only seen together ☐ a. during the mating season. ☐ b. when searching for food. ☐ c. during migrations. ☐ d. when the young need to be protected.	15	
4. The writer of this passage lives in ☐ a. America. ☐ b. England. ☐ c. Australia. ☐ d. North Africa.	15	
5. A speckled robin is ☐ a. pure white. ☐ b. striped. ☐ c. all one color. ☐ d. spotted.	15	

6. Main Idea

	Answer	Score
Mark the main idea	M	10
Mark the statement that is a detail	D	5
Mark the statement that is too narrow	N	5
Mark the statement that is too broad	B	5

a. Robins are familiar birds.

b. Robins feed their young small, green caterpillars.

c. The English found relatives of the English robin in America.

d. Robins are found throughout the world.

Total Comprehension Score
(Add your scores and enter the total on the graph on page 103.)

Categories of Comprehension Questions

No. 1: Subject Matter	No. 4: Clarifying Devices
No. 2: Supporting Details	No. 5: Vocabulary in Context
No. 3: Conclusion	No. 6: Main Idea

13. Superglue

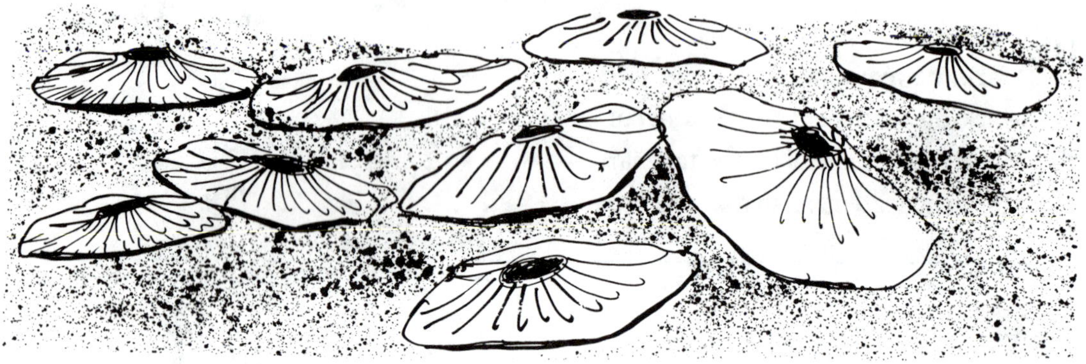

Superglue is the name I have given to barnacle cement. Barnacles stick to everything. Their Superglue is super-strong and long-lasting. Many museums have fossils of barnacles that have been glued tightly to other shells for as much as fifteen to twenty million years.

Dr. Keller tried to melt barnacle glue. He heated it to 662° Fahrenheit (about 350° Celsius) — a temperature hot enough to melt lead. The glue softened slightly, but it did not melt.

Dr. Keller didn't have any better luck when he tried to break the glue loose by freezing it. At 383° Fahrenheit (about 195° Celsius) below zero the glue still held fast. In other tests, Dr. Keller tried to dissolve the glue. Most strong acids, he found, wouldn't dissolve it. That's one reason why dentists are interested in Superglue: it won't dissolve in water.

How do barnacles make Superglue? Scientists haven't figured that out yet, but by studying how barnacles live, they are beginning to get some clues.

Newly hatched barnacles are called *larvae*. The larvae look like clams for about a week. It's during this time that they look for a place to settle down and stick tight. When they find a place — and somewhere between high and low tide with a good current and sunlight — they stop swimming and explore with their antennae.

Then a strange thing happens. Tiny drops of quick-drying Superglue appear on their antennae. Soon the animals are stuck tight.

Scientists want to find out what the glue is made of so they can make it in a laboratory. Inside the bottom of a barnacle shell, Dr. Keller found two rows of glands. One row contained a milky-white fluid that Dr. Keller thinks the barnacle uses to make its shell bigger. The glands in the other row contained a brownish fluid. Dr. Keller thinks this liquid is the Superglue!

Even though they have found the glue, the scientists' work is just beginning. They must now study it in their laboratories to find out what it is made of, and to try to make some themselves. The last step, the scientists say, could take years — or it could happen very soon.

?

	Possible Score	Your Score
1. Superglue is ☐ a. tree sap. ☐ b. beeswax. ☐ c. made by scientists. ☐ d. barnacle cement.	15	◯
2. Dr. Keller heated the glue to 662° Fahrenheit (about 350° Celsius). This is hot enough to melt ☐ a. steel. ☐ b. aluminum. ☐ c. lead. ☐ d. rock.	15	◯
3. Dentists might be interested in Superglue because it ☐ a. is a pure white color. ☐ b. is soft and easy to mold. ☐ c. will not dissolve in the mouth. ☐ d. prevents decay.	15	◯
4. The last paragraph tells us that ☐ a. Superglue is made in laboratories. ☐ b. dentists are interested in Superglue. ☐ c. Dr. Keller works with Superglue. ☐ d. scientists are still studying Superglue.	15	◯
5. A <u>fluid</u> is a ☐ a. liquid. ☐ b. gas. ☐ c. gland. ☐ d. solid.	15	◯

6. Main Idea

	Answer	Score
Mark the main idea	M	10
Mark the statement that is a detail	D	5
Mark the statement that is too narrow	N	5
Mark the statement that is too broad	B	5

a. Barnacles look like clams when they are larvae. ☐ ◯

b. Barnacles produce an extremely strong Superglue which scientists would like to copy. ☐ ◯

c. Scientists think barnacles produce their Superglue in glands under their shells. ☐ ◯

d. Barnacles can stick very tightly to their homes. ☐ ◯

Total Comprehension Score ☐
(Add your scores and enter the total on the graph on page 103.)

Categories of Comprehension Questions

No. 1: Subject Matter	No. 4: Clarifying Devices
No. 2: Supporting Details	No. 5: Vocabulary in Context
No. 3: Conclusion	No. 6: Main Idea

14. Wild Dogs of Africa

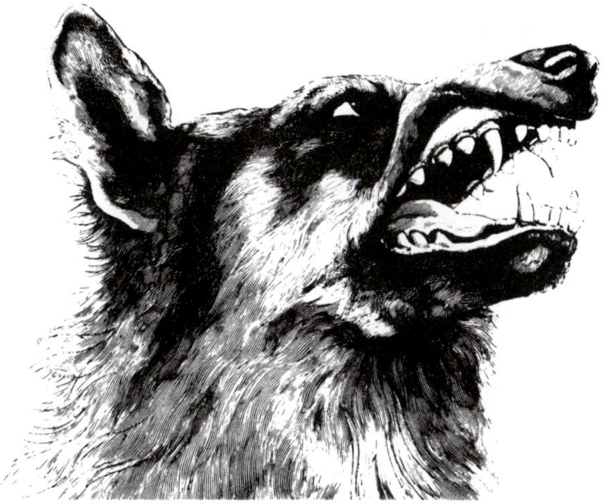

For three years I studied animals in the Serengeti National Park of East Africa. I became very interested in the life of the lion and wild dog. I watched how they both hunted such animals as antelope, zebra, and buffalo. After many days and moonlit nights, I found that their ways of life were as different as could be.

The wild dog is hated as a mean and dangerous killer of defenseless animals. It is often shot on sight just as the wolf once was in North America.

The lion, on the other hand, is "King of Beasts." People admire it for its grace and beauty. These are at least the *popular* images of these two beasts. But I found the wild dogs of Africa much more interesting to study.

Wild dogs are about the size of a setter. They have splotchy black, white and brown coats and large ears. Male and female wild dogs live together in packs made up of four to thirty animals.

A pack wanders long distances looking for food. They kill mainly those animals that are young, old or sick. All members of the pack greet and playfully chase each other before the hunt. Then they trot off to find a meal.

When a likely animal is sighted, some dogs chase it at speeds of up to forty-five miles (about 72.4 kilometers) per hour while the others move in more slowly. Often an antelope circles, and the dogs that lagged behind then swing off in a shortcut, surround the prey and attack it, ending another succesful hunt.

?

Question	Possible Score	Your Score
1. What would be another good title for this passage? ☐ a. Friends of the Wild Dog ☐ b. The Wild Dog's Way of Life ☐ c. Wild Dogs Make Good Pets ☐ d. Lazy Lions	15	
2. Wild dogs travel in a group called a ☐ a. clutch. ☐ b. flock. ☐ c. herd. ☐ d. pack.	15	
3. Wild dogs ☐ a. kill mainly for food. ☐ b. feed on dead animals they find. ☐ c. are protected by law. ☐ d. will kill mostly for sport.	15	
4. The fur of the wild dog is ☐ a. solid black. ☐ b. striped. ☐ c. gray and white. ☐ d. spotted.	15	
5. The dogs that <u>lagged</u> behind ☐ a. were the leaders. ☐ b. had poor eyesight. ☐ c. moved slowly. ☐ d. ran very fast.	15	

6. Main Idea

	Answer	Score
Mark the main idea	M	10
Mark the statement that is a detail	D	5
Mark the statement that is too narrow	N	5
Mark the statement that is too broad	B	5

a. The wild dogs greet and playfully chase each other before a hunt. ☐ ○

b. People admire lions for their grace and beauty. ☐ ○

c. Some animals which are hated have interesting lifestyles. ☐ ○

d. The author found the wild dog more interesting to study than the lion. ☐ ○

Total Comprehension Score
(Add your scores and enter the total on the graph on page 103.) ☐

Categories of Comprehension Questions

No. 1: Subject Matter	No. 4: Clarifying Devices
No. 2: Supporting Details	No. 5: Vocabulary in Context
No. 3: Conclusion	No. 6: Main Idea

15. The Hot-Cold Desert

The desert! Who would want to go to the desert — that hot, barren, sandy wasteland? That's the way many people describe the desert. But we shall see that the desert is one of the most interesting habitats on this entire planet. Once you discover its endless beauty and peace, you will want to return again and again.

Deserts are very hot because the air is so dry and clear that the sun's light comes through more strongly. In summer the sun beats down furiously. This turns the land into a radiator, which, like the radiator in your house, heats the air which touches it. One July day in Death Valley, the desert temperature went up to 134° Fahrenheit (about 57° Celsius). The land itself might be as hot as 180° Fahrenheit (about 80° Celsius). At that temperature you'd better not touch it!

But take a sweater with you when you visit the desert! Heat escapes very quickly through the mositure-free air. Soon after sunset the air cools and you will feel chilly.

Have you wondered why pictures of desert Arabs show them wearing many clothes during the hot day? Lightweight, light-colored garments insulate their bodies against heat during the day and from the cold at night.

When winter comes, many deserts are delightful places to live. Palm Springs, California, and Tucson, Arizona, are favorite winter vacation areas in the United States. Some northern or "cold" deserts, such as those in Utah and Wyoming, have plenty of cold winter weather with some snow and ice.

The desert, then, is not always hot, but it is usually dry because it gets so little rain or snow. When you are in the southern Arizona desert and you wash your hands, they almost become dry before you can reach for your towel. Sometimes when it rains only lightly, you can see the rain falling, but it disappears before it reaches the ground. The raindrops evaporate as they fall.

?

	Possible Score	Your Score
1. This passage is mostly about desert ☐ a. plants. ☐ b. animals. ☐ c. people. ☐ d. temperatures.	15	
2. The desert nights are ☐ a. windy. ☐ b. cool. ☐ c. hot. ☐ d. long.	15	
3. This passage hints that all deserts are ☐ a. hot. ☐ b. dry. ☐ c. sandy. ☐ d. wastelands.	15	
4. In the first paragraph the writer is trying to explain how most people ☐ a. live on the desert. ☐ b. enjoy the desert. ☐ c. travel on the desert. ☐ d. describe the desert.	15	
5. <u>Endless</u> beauty ☐ a. lasts forever. ☐ b. is seasonal. ☐ c. changes rapidly. ☐ d. is artificial.	15	

6. Main Idea

	Answer	Score
Mark the main idea	M	10
Mark the statement that is a detail	D	5
Mark the statement that is too narrow	N	5
Mark the statement that is too broad	B	5

a. In Death Valley, the temperature reached 134° F one day.

b. Arabs wear many garments to protect themselves from the weather.

c. The desert has changeable temperatures.

d. The desert is hot in the day and cool at night.

Total Comprehension Score
(Add your scores and enter the total on the graph on page 103.)

Categories of Comprehension Questions

No. 1: Subject Matter	No. 4: Clarifying Devices
No. 2: Supporting Details	No. 5: Vocabulary in Context
No. 3: Conclusion	No. 6: Main Idea

16. Rabies Shots

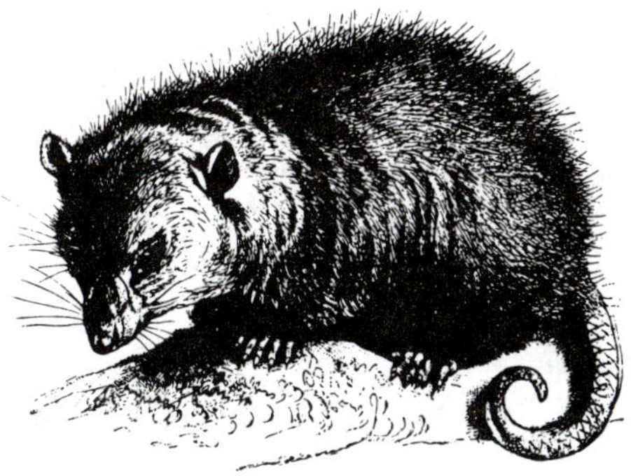

Can a pet raccoon or squirrel or possum get a rabies shot? Unfortunately, the answer is no. There is no good vaccine for captive skunks, raccoons and other wild animals, so veterinarians cannot protect them from rabies. These animals can catch rabies in their nests before they are captured and tamed. Giving those animals rabies shots later will not cure them. They can be carriers of rabies, and if they bite or scratch you, you may get the disease. The only way to know whether an animal is free from rabies is to keep it penned by itself until the veterinarian is sure it isn't infected.

Other kinds of tame animals can also carry rabies. So far, rabies vaccine has worked well on only two pets: dogs and cats. If you have a dog or cat, it must get rabies shots regularly. Usually, you get a little tag from the veterinarian to put on the collar to show the pet has been protected against rabies. If it has received its shots regularly, it won't give you rabies even if it bites you.

Much more experimenting must be done before we'll have a rabies vaccine for all furry animals. Until then, there are many kinds of cats and dogs you can have as pets — from furry kittens to big Saint Bernard dogs. You can have guppies in a fish tank or a canary in a cage. They make good pets and can live safely with humans for many years.

Foxes, raccoons, skunks, possums, squirrels, wildcats and other wild, furry animals belong in their natural homes in the woods. Leave them there and enjoy watching them — from a distance!

?

	Possible Score	Your Score
1. Humans get rabies from ☐ a. insects. ☐ b. animals. ☐ c. certain plants. ☐ d. other humans.	15	
2. So far, the rabies vaccine has worked on ☐ a. all furry animals. ☐ b. dogs and cats. ☐ c. most wild animals. ☐ d. only humans.	15	
3. The writer suggests that wild animals ☐ a. make good pets. ☐ b. are often bad-tempered. ☐ c. belong in their natural homes. ☐ d. are healthier than most pets.	15	
4. In the last paragraph the writer is trying to ☐ a. warn the reader. ☐ b. make the reader laugh. ☐ c. insult the reader. ☐ d. amuse the reader.	15	
5. If an animal is infected, it probably carries ☐ a. food. ☐ b. water. ☐ c. its young. ☐ d. disease.	15	

6. Main Idea

	Answer	Score
Mark the main idea	M	10
Mark the statement that is a detail	D	5
Mark the statement that is too narrow	N	5
Mark the statement that is too broad	B	5

a. Rabies vaccine has not entirely prevented rabies. ☐ ○

b. Rabies vaccine does not work on wild animals. ☐ ○

c. Pet raccoons, squirrels and possums can carry rabies. ☐ ○

d. Guppies and canaries are good, safe pets. ☐ ○

Total Comprehension Score ☐
(Add your scores and enter the total on the graph on page 103.)

Categories of Comprehension Questions

No. 1: Subject Matter	No. 4: Clarifying Devices
No. 2: Supporting Details	No. 5: Vocabulary in Context
No. 3: Conclusion	No. 6: Main Idea

17. The Holder of Soil and Water

Before people plowed the land, grass mixed with other plants covered much of the earth. Dead plants built up a fertile layer of soil called *humus*. A network of roots grew down into the soil. Each one made a tiny channel through which rain ran into the earth. Spongy layers of stems, leaves and roots soaked up falling rain so that it could not wash the soil away.

Then people discovered that they could plant seeds and grow crops. They began to plow the earth and remove the natural cover. The unprotected soil that had been beneath this cover blew and washed away.

Soil became damaged or *eroded* so badly that some ancient civilizations disappeared. For instance, northern Mongolia was once a rich land. But it was overgrazed by too many sheep and became a wasteland. History is full of such examples of bad land use.

In the United States, vast areas of land were plowed to make farms. The land was also overgrazed by too many cattle. Some of the land eroded so badly that it became useless. Water dug gulleys into the soil, and wind blew soil away. During the 1920s and early 1930s, soil blew away in great clouds, wiping out whole farms and burying the buildings.

After the dry years in the United States from 1925 to 1932, the whole nation became alarmed about soil erosion. So Congress set up the United States Soil Conservation Service as part of the Department of Agriculture. Scientists in this department worked with farmers and ranchers to restore the soil. They planted drainage channels with covers of living grass. They limited the number of animals that could graze on natural rangelands so the grass could grow again. And many farmers began to grow a new cover of soil-holding grass.

?

	Possible Score	Your Score
1. This passage is about ☐ a. fertilization. ☐ b. crop rotation. ☐ c. soil erosion. ☐ d. irrigation.	15	
2. The dry years in the United States came ☐ a. between 1800 and 1860. ☐ b. between 1920 and 1940. ☐ c. between 1940 and 1950. ☐ d. between 1955 and 1960.	15	
3. According to this passage, soil becomes damaged by all of the following except ☐ a. wind. ☐ b. overgrazing. ☐ c. water. ☐ d. fertilizer.	15	
4. Spongy plants ☐ a. soak up water. ☐ b. are tough. ☐ c. can be troublesome. ☐ d. bend easily.	15	
5. As used in this passage, alarmed means ☐ a. bored. ☐ b. sarcastic. ☐ c. concerned. ☐ d. useless.	15	

6. Main Idea

Mark the statement	Answer	Score
Mark the main idea	M	10
Mark the statement that is a detail	D	5
Mark the statement that is too narrow	N	5
Mark the statement that is too broad	B	5

a. We need our natural grass covers.

b. Spongy layers of stems and leaves soak up rain and hold the soil.

c. Soil unprotected by its natural cover blows or washes away.

d. Northern Mongolia was once a rich land.

Total Comprehension Score
(Add your scores and enter the total on the graph on page 103.)

Categories of Comprehension Questions

No. 1: Subject Matter	No. 4: Clarifying Devices
No. 2: Supporting Details	No. 5: Vocabulary in Context
No. 3: Conclusion	No. 6: Main Idea

18. Wild and Free

Many interesting mammals which are few in number or gone from other parts of North America can be found in abundance in Alaska.

One of these is the grizzly bear. This hump-backed, shaggy, bowlegged animal is sometimes dangerous to people, but usually it is shy and runs away when people are near. The grizzly is often called the *Alaska brown bear.* It has long been considered the world's largest land *carnivore,* or meat-eater.

The polar bear, which is also found in Alaska, grows just as large as the grizzly, but it is a sea bear. It lives on and among the ice floes of the Arctic Ocean. It sometimes visits the shores of Alaska, Canada, Greenland and Siberia.

The wolverine is another mammal that is common in Alaska, but rare or extinct in other states. It is a cousin of the mink, the otter and the weasel. The thirty-five-pound (15.9-kilogram) wolverine has stubby, powerful legs, a short tail and dark, shaggy fur. Its appetite is huge, and it will eat almost anything it can find, including mice, rabbits, birds, eggs, berries, and even fish.

Wolves roam much of Alaska. The wolf, a large member of the dog family, has long been persecuted by humans. Even in Alaska some people don't like wolves being in their areas.

Alaska also has many different kinds of hoofed mammals. One of these is the huge moose, the largest member of the deer family. There are also caribou, musk ox, elk and the tiny Sitka black-tailed deer.

Other hoofed mammals of Alaska include the white Dall sheep and white mountain goats which live in Alaska's high mountains. They are not really goats, but a kind of antelope, with soft pads on the bottoms of the hoofs that help them stick to rocks on steep mountain slopes.

Today Alaska's mammals exist mostly undisturbed by humans — but how long will it last?

?

	Possible Score	Your Score
1. This passage is about ☐ a. reptiles in Alaska. ☐ b. the Alaskan king crab. ☐ c. mammals of Alaska. ☐ d. birds of Alaska.	15	
2. Which of the following is considered the world's largest meat-eating animal? ☐ a. Wolverine ☐ b. Grizzly bear ☐ c. Polar bear ☐ d. Caribou	15	
3. From this passage, we can guess that animals may become few in number or extinct because of ☐ a. people. ☐ b. disease. ☐ c. lack of water. ☐ d. too little food.	15	
4. The grizzly bear is described as ☐ a. having a short tail and shaggy fur. ☐ b. a member of the gorilla family. ☐ c. a plant eater. ☐ d. hump-backed, shaggy, and bowlegged.	15	
5. In this passage, <u>persecuted</u> means ☐ a. helped. ☐ b. hunted down. ☐ c. enjoyed. ☐ d. taken care of.	15	

6. Main Idea

	Answer	Score
Mark the main idea	M	10
Mark the statement that is a detail	D	5
Mark the statement that is too narrow	N	5
Mark the statement that is too broad	B	5

a. The grizzly, now rare in the lower United States, is abundant in Alaska.

b. The wolverine has a huge appetite.

c. Many of the animals now rare in the lower United States are plentiful in Alaska.

d. Safe places for animals are getting fewer.

Total Comprehension Score
(Add your scores and enter the total on the graph on page 103.)

Categories of Comprehension Questions

No. 1: Subject Matter	No. 4: Clarifying Devices
No. 2: Supporting Details	No. 5: Vocabulary in Context
No. 3: Conclusion	No. 6: Main Idea

19. The Horse of the Bedouins

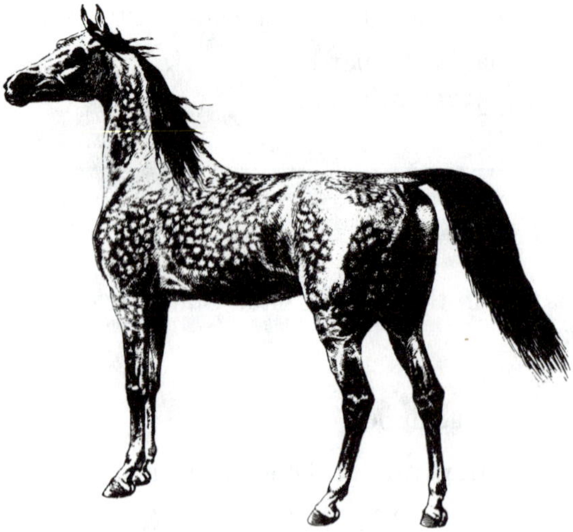

The Arabian horse is a beautiful animal. Some say the most beautiful in all the world. It has an intelligent head and alert eyes. Its beauty can be seen in its pointed ears, high arching neck and flowing mane. And when it moves, its floating gait is poetry itself brought to life.

Yet, in the early part of this century, its very beauty made it an unpopular animal in the United States. It was *too* beautiful for work. It was not even a good horse for "show." It was too small. For show, people like the large, flashy saddle horse whose high-stepping gait and upraised tail bring the spectators to their feet cheering. Then, suddenly, this intelligent, beautiful and gentle horse captured the hearts of horse lovers in the United States. Now, in one state alone, California, there are more Arabian horses than in all of Arabia.

The Bedouins of the desert say that God created their horse out of the wind and gave it to them as their most prized possession. And the Bedouins treat the horse well. It even sleeps in the tent of its owner at night. It is ready for instant action in case of danger. It is ready to signal danger by whinnying or stamping its feet.

In truth, the Bedouins could not have survived in the deep, huge, sandy desert without the Arabian horse's toughness, strength of endurance and ability to survive on a small amount of food. In war, it could run circles around other cavalry horses. Truly, the Arabian is the horse of the Bedouins. They need it and they love it.

?

	Possible Score	Your Score
1. This passage tells us ☐ a. many facts about Arabian horses. ☐ b. all about Arab tribes. ☐ c. about the kinds of Arabian horses. ☐ d. about United States horses.	15	
2. Which state has more Arabian horses than Arabia itself does? ☐ a. Texas ☐ b. Colorado ☐ c. Oklahoma ☐ d. California	15	
3. The Bedouins consider their horses to be ☐ a. a weak breed. ☐ b. a means of income. ☐ c. something very special. ☐ d. work horses.	15	
4. An Arabian horse can "run circles around other cavalry horses." This means that Arabian horses ☐ a. attack by running in circles. ☐ b. will not mix with cavalry horses. ☐ c. run in the opposite direction of cavalry horses. ☐ d. can run faster and longer then cavalry horses.	15	
5. What is a horse's gait? ☐ a. The way a horse steps ☐ b. Its flowing mane ☐ c. The high arching neck ☐ d. Its pointed ears	15	

6. Main Idea

	Answer	Score
Mark the main idea	M	10
Mark the statement that is a detail	D	5
Mark the statement that is too narrow	N	5
Mark the statement that is too broad	B	5

a. The saddle horse is large and flashy.

b. Some horses are very special.

c. The Arabian horse sleeps in the tent of its Bedouin owners.

d. The Arabian horse is a beautiful animal beloved by many.

Total Comprehension Score
(Add your scores and enter the total on the graph on page 103.)

Categories of Comprehension Questions

No. 1: Subject Matter	No. 4: Clarifying Devices
No. 2: Supporting Details	No. 5: Vocabulary in Context
No. 3: Conclusion	No. 6: Main Idea

20. Delightful Dolphins

A few years ago Milton Santini was a fisherman. Now he makes his living by catching dolphins. It all began several years ago when Milt and his brother, natives of Florida, were fishing off the Florida Keys. As they were heading home they noticed a dolphin following them. The dolphin frolicked and splashed around their boat. Milt remarked to his brother, "Why, it's so friendly — I bet I can catch it with my hands." So Milt decided to see what he could do. Before very long he brought the dolphin aboard. Now Milt was eager to get home to show his wife, Ginny, their unusual new pet. They bought wire fencing and made a sea pool in the inlet next to their home. At the time they didn't know that this would lead them into a new and unusual career.

Ginny helped Milt in his new work. Each time they went hunting, she held the net beside the boat and slowly pulled it in while Milt was in the water talking gently to the dolphin and coaxing it to come aboard.

Once the dolphin was aboard, Ginny put a cloth cover on it. She had made it to protect the dolphin from the hot sun until it was safe in its new sea pool. There it would be fed and protected from the dangers of the sea.

The dolphins enjoyed playing and being near people in their new home. Sometimes a dolphin would jump into the ocean, but it always returned to its friends at the Santinis' sea pool.

Each day Milt and Ginny discovered more about the intelligent and mischievous ways of their dolphins. It was Ginny who first started swimming with their favorite dolphin named Mitzi. By holding onto Mitzi's dorsal fin, she could go for a thrilling ride in the salty water. A movie company heard about Mitzi and decided to use her in a movie called *Flipper*.

Word traveled to neighboring towns. Soon Milt was getting letters and phone calls from sea aquariums, zoos and marinelands. Scientists wanted dolphins so they could learn more about their behavior.

Mealtime became a kind of training game. For each effort a dolphin made in learning a new trick, a fish dinner was its reward. Now people were coming every day at mealtime to watch the funny antics of the dolphins. So Milt and Ginny decided to have a dolphin show and charge admission.

?

	Possible Score	Your Score
1. This passage is about ☐ a. dangerous dolphins. ☐ b. dolphins used for scientific experiments. ☐ c. a newly discovered species of dolphin. ☐ d. pet dolphins.	15	
2. This passage takes place in ☐ a. Mississippi. ☐ b. California. ☐ c. Texas. ☐ d. Florida.	15	
3. Milt and Ginny ☐ a. did not plan on a career in dolphin training. ☐ b. studied long and hard in order to raise dolphins. ☐ c. were oceanographers. ☐ d. have always wanted to train dolphins.	15	
4. Dolphins can be described as ☐ a. fearsome. ☐ b. quarrelsome. ☐ c. playful. ☐ d. unkind.	15	
5. A good synonym for <u>antic</u> is ☐ a. prank. ☐ b. fin. ☐ c. noise. ☐ d. appearance.	15	

6. Main Idea

	Answer	Score
Mark the main idea	M	10
Mark the statement that is a detail	D	5
Mark the statement that is too narrow	N	5
Mark the statement that is too broad	B	5

a. Dolphins can be trained to do tricks if rewarded with fish. ☐ ○

b. A movie called *Flipper* was made using a dolphin. ☐ ○

c. Milt and Ginny found a way to catch and train dolphins. ☐ ○

d. People in Florida can catch dolphins. ☐ ○

Total Comprehension Score ☐
(Add your scores and enter the total on the graph on page 103.)

Categories of Comprehension Questions

No. 1: Subject Matter	No. 4: Clarifying Devices
No. 2: Supporting Details	No. 5: Vocabulary in Context
No. 3: Conclusion	No. 6: Main Idea

21. The Fighting Bass

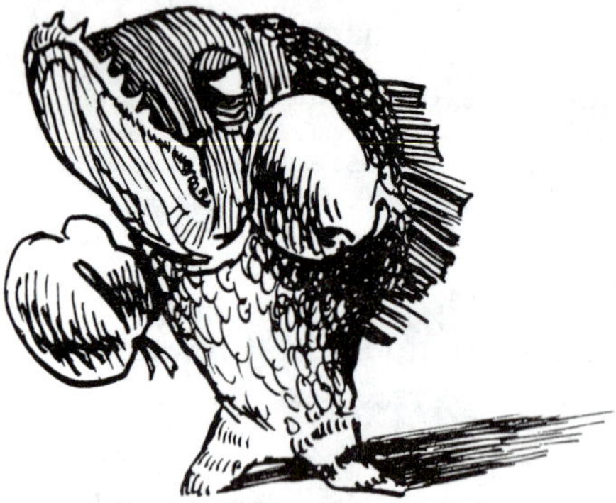

Every day, for all the animals below the still waters of a peaceful lake, there is a life and death struggle going on. Each animal, whether big or small, is living its own life cycle. An animal is born, develops movement, learns to catch food, mates and sometimes dies naturally of old age.

More often, however, it becomes food for another animal. Thus, not all the animals complete their life cycles because animal life is *interdependent.* That is, life lives off other life. Sometimes an animal is the hunter and at other times, the prey.

The largemouth bass is found in many freshwater lakes in this country. Whether in dark depths or sunny shallow water, weedy swamp or upland stream, the largemouth bass is known to be one of the smartest game fish.

The life cycle of the bass starts in the spring. The spawning male bass heads for shallow water, and there he clears an area for a nest. He uses his tail to fan the lake bed and remove all loose sand and particles until the grass roots in the lake bottom appear.

A female bass joins him. She is usually much larger than the male. When the clearing is finished, the female lays her eggs and the male fertilizes them.

Then the male takes over protecting the eggs. He even chases the female away from the nest, for females often eat their own eggs. When his nest is threatened, he will attack an enemy many times his size. Sunfish and other fish can "smell" the eggs and rush in to eat them. Often, while the bass is busy chasing one sunfish away, another sunfish rushes in and helps itself to the eggs.

?

Question	Possible Score	Your Score
1. This passage mostly talks about ☐ a. different kinds of fresh water fish. ☐ b. bass fishing. ☐ c. the life cycle of the bass. ☐ d. stocking fresh water lakes.	15	
2. Female bass ☐ a. often eat their own eggs. ☐ b. feed on sunfish. ☐ c. fertilize the eggs. ☐ d. are smaller than the male.	15	
3. Many animals never die of old age because ☐ a. animals never age. ☐ b. most of the time they die of disease. ☐ c. they are usually killed by another animal. ☐ d. animals have strong hearts.	15	
4. A "weedy" swamp is filled with many ☐ a. insects. ☐ b. animals. ☐ c. plants. ☐ d. rocks.	15	
5. When a nest is threatened it is ☐ a. not well built. ☐ b. untidy. ☐ c. well made. ☐ d. in danger.	15	

6. Main Idea

	Answer	Score
Mark the main idea	M	10
Mark the statement that is a detail	D	5
Mark the statement that is too narrow	N	5
Mark the statement that is too broad	B	5

a. There is a life and death struggle going on in ponds. ☐ ○

b. The male bass protects the eggs. ☐ ○

c. In the life cycle of the bass, a large, freshwater game fish, the male builds the nest and protects the eggs. ☐ ○

d. The female bass is usually larger than the male. ☐ ○

Total Comprehension Score ☐
(Add your scores and enter the total on the graph on page 103.)

Categories of Comprehension Questions

No. 1: Subject Matter	No. 4: Clarifying Devices
No. 2: Supporting Details	No. 5: Vocabulary in Context
No. 3: Conclusion	No. 6: Main Idea

22. Utterly Ridiculous

When people exploring Australia discovered the platypus in the early 1800s, they sent skins and descriptions of the funny animal back to Europe. Animal experts from many nations saw this strange new animal and began to quarrel about it. "An animal with fur and webbed feet and a bill like a duck's! Impossible!" some said. "A mammal which lays eggs! Ridiculous!" said others.

These educated people just couldn't believe such an animal really existed. It couldn't be a reptile because it was warm-blooded. It couldn't be a mammal because it laid eggs. It couldn't be a bird because it had no wings or feathers. Some even said they were being tricked — that the platypus didn't exist at all. But they were wrong. The platypus lived then, and it lives today to amaze us all. It is one of two known mammals in the whole world which breed their young by laying eggs!

This furry little animal is about twenty inches (about 50.8 centimeters) long. Its tail is long and flat, something like a beaver's. It has a broad, flat bill like a duck's — in fact, the platypus is called a *duckbill.*

Another interesting thing about this shy, little animal is that it spends a lot of its time in the water as well as on land. It is *semiaquatic.* Morning and evening it goes into water to find food on the bottoms of streams. It may dive underwater and stay under for as long as five minutes while searching for worms, the eggs of water insects, tiny shelled animals and small fish. Although the platypus has keen eyesight and hearing on land, it is completely blind and deaf underwater because it covers its eyes and ears with folds of skin to keep the water out. Only a highly developed sense of touch in its bill guides it to food.

Now, don't you agree that the platypus must have been very confusing to the people who first discovered it? But wait. This fascinating little creature has more surprises in store for you. When it is in the water, it has webbed feet like a duck's to help it swim. When it returns to dry land, it folds back the webs to uncover claws on its front feet. These claws help it walk and dig burrows!

Even today, mystery surrounds the amazing platypus despite all that modern science has learned about it. The male platypus, for example, has two poison-filled spurs on his rear legs, but no one knows why. Some people think he uses them to kill his rivals in the lovers' duel for a mate, but that is just a guess.

?

	Possible Score	Your Score
1. The platypus is ☐ a. a mammal. ☐ b. a reptile. ☐ c. a bird. ☐ d. an amphibian.	15	
2. The platypus was discovered in the ☐ a. early 1800s. ☐ b. middle 1800s. ☐ c. late 1800s. ☐ d. early 1900s.	15	
3. This passage leads us to believe that most mammals ☐ a. live in the water. ☐ b. have fur. ☐ c. are cold blooded. ☐ d. do not lay eggs.	15	
4. How did some early scientists first feel about the platypus? ☐ a. They were afraid of it. ☐ b. They were bored with it. ☐ c. They were sure it did not exist. ☐ d. They disliked it.	15	
5. As used in this passage, a rival is ☐ a. a neighbor. ☐ b. an enemy. ☐ c. a mate. ☐ d. a friend.	15	

6. Main Idea

	Answer	Score
Mark the main idea	M	10
Mark the statement that is a detail	D	5
Mark the statement that is too narrow	N	5
Mark the statement that is too broad	B	5

a. The platypus was discovered in Australia in the 1800s.

b. Mystery and amazement surround the platypus.

c. The platypus is truly a most unusual animal.

d. The platypus is unusual because it is a mammal yet it lays eggs.

Total Comprehension Score
(Add your scores and enter the total on the graph on page 103.)

Categories of Comprehension Questions

No. 1: Subject Matter	No. 4: Clarifying Devices
No. 2: Supporting Details	No. 5: Vocabulary in Context
No. 3: Conclusion	No. 6: Main Idea

23. What a Life

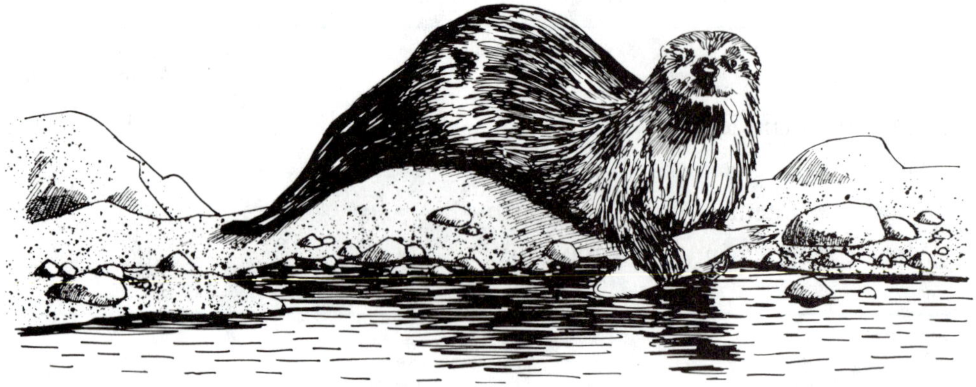

Since wild otters are seldom seen, most of what we know about them comes from studies made by people who, by purest accident, picked up and raised wild babies just for the fun of it and then found themselves enslaved for life by their inexpressible charm. Such wild baby otters mature into domesticated, not captive, animals — an important distinction.

From people who have studied them, here are some facts. They are long-lived — ten to twenty years and more. They are prodigiously active. Their intense curiosity gets them into constant trouble. They tend to group in a single small family or to go it alone. They are great travelers by water, partly in search of food or to find a mate and partly, perhaps, for the change of scenery.

Otters love crawfish, frogs, turtles, water snakes and worms. Occasionally they will eat a muskrat or a coot or a duck — even a Canada goose. Underwater, they use their long whiskers as feelers to warn them of obstructions or of the nippers of crustaceans.

They do not hibernate in winter but nobody ever sees them then. They stay out of sight in tree root hollows or in burrows that they have appropriated from other animals and enlarged. Such an otter burrow is reached from below the water level of a stream by an inclined tunnel that may be as long as fifty feet (about 15.2 meters).

Birth takes place in the dead of winter. The northern mother protects the babies from the cold by curling her body completely around them. She takes her own good time bringing them up. Meanwhile, she requires that the father keep his distance — at least a half-mile (about .8 kilometers). He can stop to look briefly now and then, but he may not get familiar with his children.

At birth, otter cubs are the size of small chipmunks. They are born blind and do not open their eyes until a month has passed. After two months, the mother weans them on small frogs and worms. At three months, she coaxes them into the water to learn to swim or pushes them in if they hesitate. She continues her tutoring through the summer and fall. She does not cast them out into the world until just before preparing her burrow for the arrival of a new brood.

?

	Possible Score	Your Score
1. The topic under discussion in this passage is ☐ a. the otter's burrow. ☐ b. the wild otter's diet. ☐ c. wild otter behavior. ☐ d. fashionable uses of otter fur.	15	
2. Otters are ☐ a. meat eaters. ☐ b. vegetarians. ☐ c. carion eaters. ☐ d. insectivores.	15	
3. Who raises the young otters? ☐ a. The female ☐ b. The male ☐ c. Both male and female ☐ d. Young otters care for themselves.	15	
4. Underwater the otter uses its whiskers for ☐ a. touching. ☐ b. hearing. ☐ c. seeing. ☐ d. smelling.	15	
5. To enlarge means ☐ a. to bury. ☐ b. to cover up. ☐ c. to make bigger. ☐ d. to abandon.	15	

6. Main Idea

	Answer	Score
Mark the main idea	M	10
Mark the statement that is a detail	D	5
Mark the statement that is too narrow	N	5
Mark the statement that is too broad	B	5

a. People who have raised them say that otters are very active.

b. Facts about the otter come mostly from people who have raised them.

c. We don't know much about wild otters.

d. Otters love to eat crawfish.

Total Comprehension Score
(Add your scores and enter the total on the graph on page 103.)

Categories of Comprehension Questions

No. 1: Subject Matter	No. 4: Clarifying Devices
No. 2: Supporting Details	No. 5: Vocabulary in Context
No. 3: Conclusion	No. 6: Main Idea

24. Save the Giant

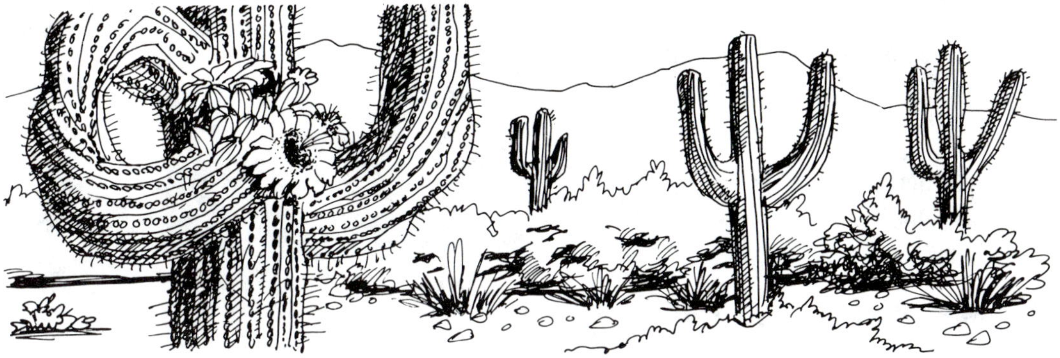

The white-winged dove visits the saguaro forests where it feeds on the flowers and fruit. In so doing it covers its face and body with the yellow pollen. Then the pollen gets spread from one blossom to another, helping to pollinate the cacti.

The saguaro's life is threatened mostly by two enemies — humans and disease. Even though it is a thirty-foot (about 9.1-meter) giant weighing ten tons (about 9 tonnes), people can kill it in an instant. But why would anyone want to kill such a handsome plant? Unfortunately, persons we call vandals think it is fun to destroy things. They drive up to a saguaro cactus and push it over with their automobile bumper. In one second they destroy a desert giant that has lived in peace for perhaps 150 years or more. Other vandals "stab" saguaros by throwing sharp stones at them just to see the stones stick in the fleshy covering. This weakens the plants and allows bacteria to enter. Some persons prefer to shoot holes in the giant plants, but the effects are the same. The saguaro is doomed when any of these things is done to it.

Have you heard stories about how people dying of thirst have gotten water from the saguaro as they might from a big jug? The stories are not true. Saguaros do store water, but there is no juglike cavity inside the plant. Its liquid is held in the same way as the juice inside a melon. But saguaro juice is like glue and has a bad taste. It will irritate your throat and actually make you more thirsty. By storing water in its own body, a saguaro can live for two years without rain. When a drought lasts a long time, though, weak and diseased cacti often die.

Just the same, some persons are not satisfied until they have cut down a saguaro and found this out for themselves. Others chop down the plants just to see what they look like inside.

The saguaro has natural enemies, too. A little moth carries bacteria from one saguaro to another and this kills some of the cactuses. Rodents, moths and the hot sun destroy many young saguaros. These are nature's ways of keeping saguaros from becoming too numerous.

Saguaros have been successful in surviving for millions of years, far longer than humans have lived on earth. Let's not be among those who destroy this giant of plants.

?

	Possible Score	Your Score
1. This passage is about a giant ☐ a. tree. ☐ b. whale. ☐ c. cactus. ☐ d. squid.	15	
2. The giant saguaro may weigh as much as ☐ a. 2 tons. ☐ b. 4 tons. ☐ c. 7 tons. ☐ d. 10 tons.	15	
3. Which of the following is most likely true? ☐ a. The saguaro can store water for long periods of time. ☐ b. Saguaros are becoming too numerous. ☐ c. Saguaro juice is very tasty. ☐ d. Many stories have been written about the saguaro's life.	15	
4. The juice of the saguaro is like glue. This means it is ☐ a. harmful. ☐ b. good to eat. ☐ c. sticky. ☐ d. hot.	15	
5. As used in this passage a cavity is ☐ a. a small scratch. ☐ b. harmful germs. ☐ c. fleshy skin. ☐ d. a hollow space.	15	

6. Main Idea

	Answer	Score
Mark the main idea	M	10
Mark the statement that is a detail	D	5
Mark the statement that is too narrow	N	5
Mark the statement that is too broad	B	5

a. The two worst enemies of the saguaro are humans and disease.

b. The saguaros in our deserts are being destroyed.

c. Healthy saguaros live over 150 years.

d. Through vandalism, humans destroy many saguaros.

Total Comprehension Score
(Add your scores and enter the total on the graph on page 103.)

Categories of Comprehension Questions

No. 1: Subject Matter	No. 4: Clarifying Devices
No. 2: Supporting Details	No. 5: Vocabulary in Context
No. 3: Conclusion	No. 6: Main Idea

25. The Ocelot

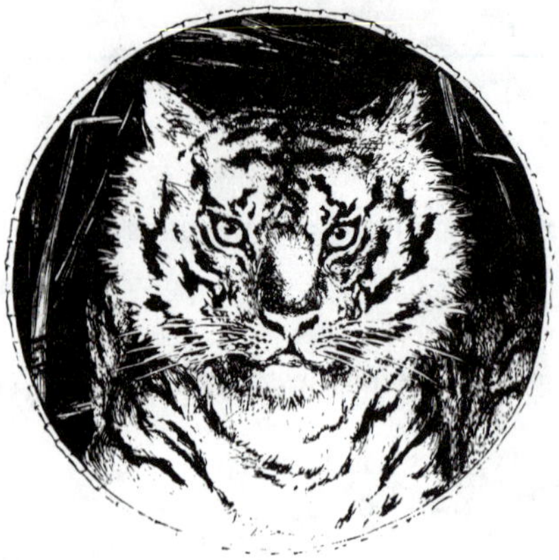

The ocelot has a face and head striped like a tiger's. The rest of its body is covered with spots like a leopard. It can be found from southern Texas and Arizona through Mexico and into much of South America.

The ocelot usually hunts in the evening and at night, but it may hunt during the day if it is very hungry. As the cat searches the forest, its large, reddish-brown eyes are alert for anything it can catch and kill — rats, mice, agoutis, monkeys and birds. It will even eat frogs and snakes. It may do a bit of fishing as well, for it is a good swimmer.

Ocelot kittens are born in the fall or early winter. The mother gives birth in a cave or rocky den, or sometimes in a hollow tree. Unlike many cats, male ocelots usually stay with their mates and help raise the young.

Ocelots have few natural enemies. The big jaguar may make a meal of an ocelot now and then. Sometimes large eagles carry off a small cat or kitten. But humans are the ocelot's most dangerous enemy.

The ocelot's beautiful coat makes it the target of skin hunters. Natives shoot and trap ocelots by the thousands and sell them to fur dealers. Many South American and Central American countries now have laws against selling ocelot skins. But often they do not enforce the laws.

If all the laws were enforced, the lovely ocelot might have a chance. But the ocelot also needs large parts of the jungle set aside as national parks and sanctuaries, where it and other animals can live safely.

?

	Possible Score	Your Score
1. The ocelot is a type of ☐ a. water bird. ☐ b. wild dog. ☐ c. rodent. ☐ d. cat.	15	
2. The ocelot lives in ☐ a. Texas, Arizona, Mexico and South America. ☐ b. Africa and India. ☐ c. Washington, Oregon and Canada. ☐ d. areas throughout the entire North American continent.	15	
3. After the young are born, most male cats ☐ a. do not stay with their families. ☐ b. feed the babies. ☐ c. help raise the young. ☐ d. are also cared for by the female.	15	
4. The ocelot's coat can be described as ☐ a. attractive. ☐ b. common. ☐ c. ugly. ☐ d. useless.	15	
5. An alert ocelot is one which is ☐ a. lazy. ☐ b. strong. ☐ c. blind. ☐ d. watchful.	15	

6. Main Idea

	Answer	Score
Mark the main idea	M	10
Mark the statement that is a detail	D	5
Mark the statement that is too narrow	N	5
Mark the statement that is too broad	B	5

a. Humans are the ocelot's enemy.

b. Ocelot skins are sold to fur dealers.

c. Ocelots eat monkeys and snakes.

d. The ocelot is hunted by humans for its skin.

Total Comprehension Score
(Add your scores and enter the total on the graph on page 103.)

Categories of Comprehension Questions

No. 1: Subject Matter	No. 4: Clarifying Devices
No. 2: Supporting Details	No. 5: Vocabulary in Context
No. 3: Conclusion	No. 6: Main Idea

Acknowledgments

The passages appearing in this book have been reprinted with the kind permission of the following publications and publishers to whom the author is indebted:

Aramco World Magazine, published by The Arabian American Oil Company, New York, New York.

The Communicator, published by the New York State Outdoor Education Association, Syracuse, New York.

The Conservationist, published by the New York State Conservation Department, Albany, New York.

A Cornell Science Leaflet, published by the New York State College of Agriculture and Life Sciences, a unit of the State University, at Cornell University, Ithaca, New York.

Food, The Yearbook of Agriculture, published by the United States Department of Agriculture, Washington, D.C.

Handbook of Nature-Study, published by Comstock Publishing Company, Ithaca, New York.

Kansas Fish & Game, published by the Kansas Forestry, Fish and Game Commission, Pratt, Kansas.

National Wildlife, published by The National Wildlife Federation, Washington, D.C.

Outdoor Oklahoma, published by the Oklahoma Department of Wildlife Conservation, Oklahoma City, Oklahoma.

Pennsylvania Game News, published by the Pennsylvania Game Commission, Harrisburg, Pennsylvania.

Ranger Rick's Nature Magazine, published by The National Wildlife Federation, Washington, D.C.

The Tennessee Conservationist, published by the Tennessee Department of Conservation and the Tennessee Game and Fish Commission.

Answer Key: Book 10

Passage 1:	1.**a**	2.**a**	3.**b**	4.**d**	5.**b**	6a.**M**	6b.**N**	6c.**D**	6d.**B**
Passage 2:	1.**c**	2.**c**	3.**c**	4.**b**	5.**d**	6a.**D**	6b.**M**	6c.**N**	6d.**B**
Passage 3:	1.**d**	2.**a**	3.**b**	4.**d**	5.**b**	6a.**N**	6b.**M**	6c.**D**	6d.**B**
Passage 4:	1.**b**	2.**d**	3.**a**	4.**d**	5.**c**	6a.**B**	6b.**M**	6c.**N**	6d.**D**
Passage 5:	1.**c**	2.**d**	3.**b**	4.**d**	5.**a**	6a.**M**	6b.**N**	6c.**D**	6d.**B**
Passage 6:	1.**a**	2.**b**	3.**d**	4.**d**	5.**a**	6a.**B**	6b.**N**	6c.**M**	6d.**D**
Passage 7:	1.**b**	2.**a**	3.**c**	4.**b**	5.**d**	6a.**B**	6b.**D**	6c.**M**	6d.**N**
Passage 8:	1.**b**	2.**d**	3.**a**	4.**d**	5.**b**	6a.**B**	6b.**N**	6c.**M**	6d.**D**
Passage 9:	1.**d**	2.**b**	3.**a**	4.**c**	5.**c**	6a.**M**	6b.**N**	6c.**D**	6d.**B**
Passage 10:	1.**c**	2.**d**	3.**c**	4.**b**	5.**d**	6a.**D**	6b.**B**	6c.**M**	6d.**N**
Passage 11:	1.**b**	2.**a**	3.**c**	4.**a**	5.**c**	6a.**D**	6b.**N**	6c.**B**	6d.**M**
Passage 12:	1.**c**	2.**b**	3.**a**	4.**b**	5.**d**	6a.**B**	6b.**D**	6c.**N**	6d.**M**
Passage 13:	1.**d**	2.**c**	3.**c**	4.**d**	5.**a**	6a.**D**	6b.**M**	6c.**N**	6d.**B**

Passage 14:	1.**b**	2.**d**	3.**a**	4.**d**	5.**c**	6a.**N**	6b.**D**	6c.**B**	6d.**M**
Passage 15:	1.**d**	2.**b**	3.**b**	4.**d**	5.**a**	6a.**N**	6b.**D**	6c.**B**	6d.**M**
Passage 16:	1.**b**	2.**b**	3.**c**	4.**a**	5.**d**	6a.**B**	6b.**M**	6c.**N**	6d.**D**
Passage 17:	1.**c**	2.**b**	3.**d**	4.**a**	5.**c**	6a.**B**	6b.**N**	6c.**M**	6d.**D**
Passage 18:	1.**c**	2.**b**	3.**a**	4.**d**	5.**b**	6a.**N**	6b.**D**	6c.**M**	6d.**B**
Passage 19:	1.**a**	2.**d**	3.**c**	4.**d**	5.**a**	6a.**D**	6b.**B**	6c.**N**	6d.**M**
Passage 20:	1.**d**	2.**d**	3.**a**	4.**c**	5.**a**	6a.**N**	6b.**D**	6c.**M**	6d.**B**
Passage 21:	1.**c**	2.**a**	3.**c**	4.**c**	5.**d**	6a.**B**	6b.**N**	6c.**M**	6d.**D**
Passage 22:	1.**a**	2.**a**	3.**d**	4.**c**	5.**b**	6a.**D**	6b.**B**	6c.**M**	6d.**N**
Passage 23:	1.**c**	2.**a**	3.**a**	4.**a**	5.**c**	6a.**N**	6b.**M**	6c.**B**	6d.**D**
Passage 24:	1.**c**	2.**d**	3.**a**	4.**c**	5.**d**	6a.**M**	6b.**B**	6c.**D**	6d.**N**
Passage 25:	1.**d**	2.**a**	3.**a**	4.**a**	5.**d**	6a.**B**	6b.**N**	6c.**D**	6d.**M**

Diagnostic Chart (For Student Correction)

Directions: Write your final answers in the *upper* part of the passage block. Then correct your answers using the Answer Key on pages 100 and 101. If your answer is correct, do not make any more marks in the block. If your answer is incorrect, write the letter of the correct answer in the *lower* part of the block.

Categories of Comprehension Skills		Reading Passage 1	2	3	4	5	6	7	8	9	10	11	12	13	14	15	16	17	18	19	20	21	22	23	24	25
1. Subject Matter																										
2. Supporting Details																										
3. Conclusion																										
4. Clarifying Devices																										
5. Vocabulary in Context																										
6. Main Idea	Main Idea																									
	Detail																									
	Too Narrow																									
	Too Broad																									

Progress Graph

Directions: Write your Total Comprehension Score in the box under the number for each passage. Then put an *x* along the line above each box to show your Total Comprehension Score for that passage. Then make a graph of your progress. Draw a line to connect the *x*'s.

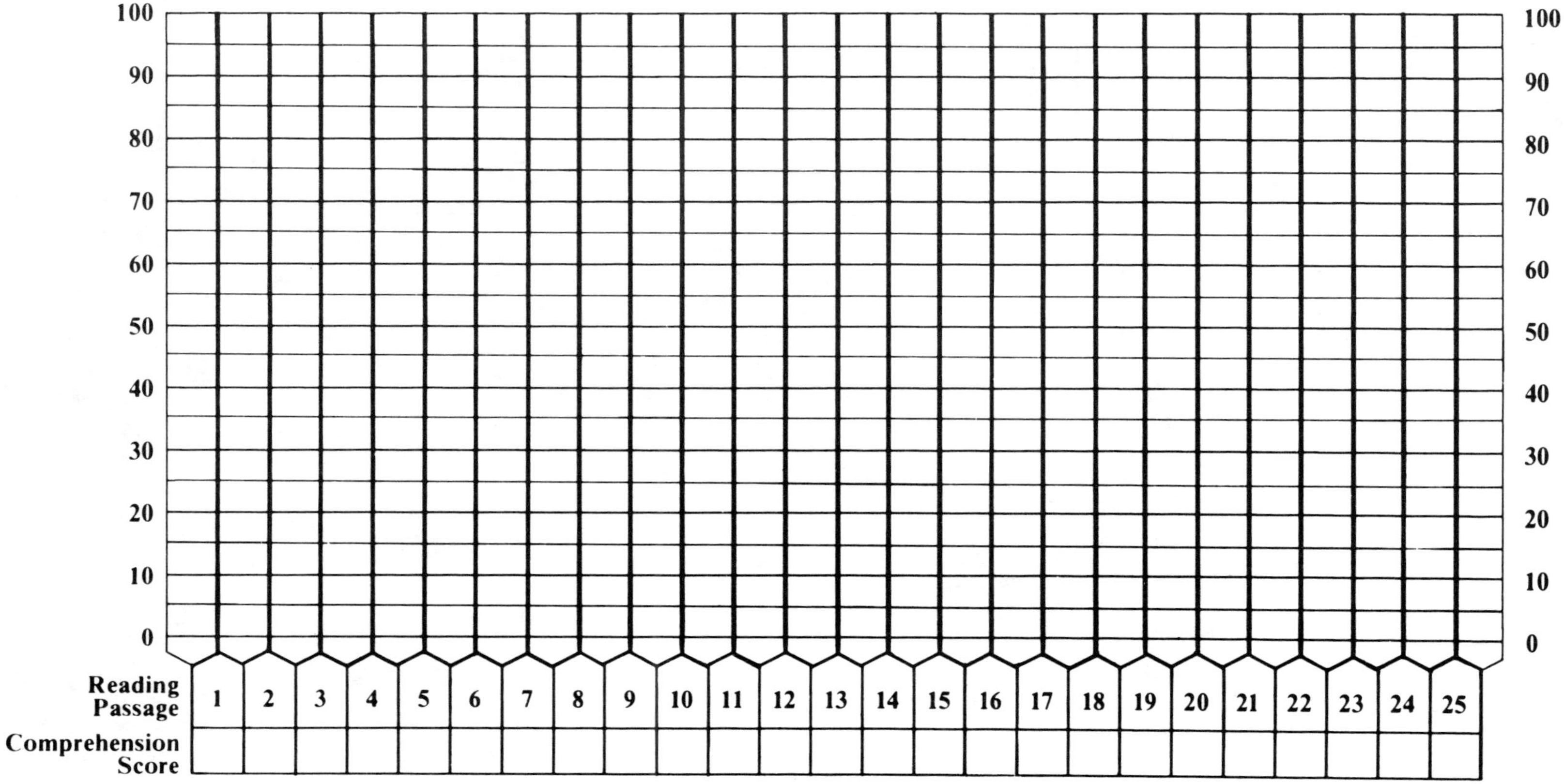

Classroom Management System

Classroom Management System
(For Teacher Correction)

To the Teacher

The Classroom Management System provides an easy and effective way to individualize instruction. It can be used by reading specialists as well as by regular classroom teachers. The management system is designed to be equally effective when used with a single student, a small group, or a full-size class.

The Classroom Management System provides ongoing assessment of student work for both you and your student. It shows not only the amount of work completed, but also the quality of the work.

It serves as a diagnostic tool by revealing patterns of errors at a glance. For example, if a student has difficulty identifying subject matter (question #1 in each set of questions throughout the *Essential Skills Series*), a pattern of errors will appear in the Subject Matter column of the Classroom Management System Record Sheet. This will enable you to focus on the specific skills needs of each student.

The Classroom Management System Record Sheet is on pages 108-109. Both pages may be duplicated and stapled together.

How to Use the Classroom Management System Record Sheet

Step 1: Have the student answer the questions for each *Essential Skills* passage under the appropriate question heading.

Passage	① Subject Matter	② Supporting Details	③ Conclusion	④ Clarifying Devices	⑤ Vocabulary in Context	⑥ Main Idea				Number Correct	Errors Corrected
						a	b	c	d		
1	d	c	a	b	d	N	D	B	M		

Step 2: Circle any incorrect answers and fill in the total number correct.

1	d	c (circled)	a	b	d	N (circled)	D (circled)	B	M	6	

Step 3: Have the student correct his or her incorrect answers.

1	d	c b	a	b	d	D/N	N/D	B	M		

Step 4: Give assistance as needed and, if necessary, correct the student's adjusted answers.

1	d	c b	a	b	d	D/N	N/D	B	M	6	

Step 5: Have the student go on to the next passage.

2	b	b	a	d	a	M	B	N	D	6	✓

Step 6: Repeat Steps 1-4. If the class is large, it may be necessary to have students complete two or three passages before you correct them. This will slow the "traffic" at your desk.

Note: It is important for students to analyze and, to the extent possible, correct their own errors (Step 3).

Essential Skills Series

Classroom Management System **Record Sheet**

(For Teacher Correction)

Name ______________________

Teacher ______________________

Date ______________________

Book Number ______________________

To the Student: Write your answers in the spaces provided. (See the Example below.) Your teacher will circle any incorrect answers. Then go back over the questions and correct your mistakes.

Passage	① Subject Matter	② Supporting Details	③ Conclusion	④ Clarifying Devices	⑤ Vocabulary in Context	⑥ Main Idea a	b	c	d	Number Correct	Errors Corrected
Example	c	(b) a	d	a	c	D (N)	N (D)	M	B		
1											
2											
3											
4											
5											
6											
7											
8											
9											
10											

Name ______________________ Book No.__________ Classroom Management System Record Sheet

	1	2	3	4	5	6					
11											
12											
13											
14											
15											
16											
17											
18											
19											
20											
21											
22											
23											
24											
25											